Correlative Neuroanatomy of Computed Tomography and Magnetic Resonance Imaging

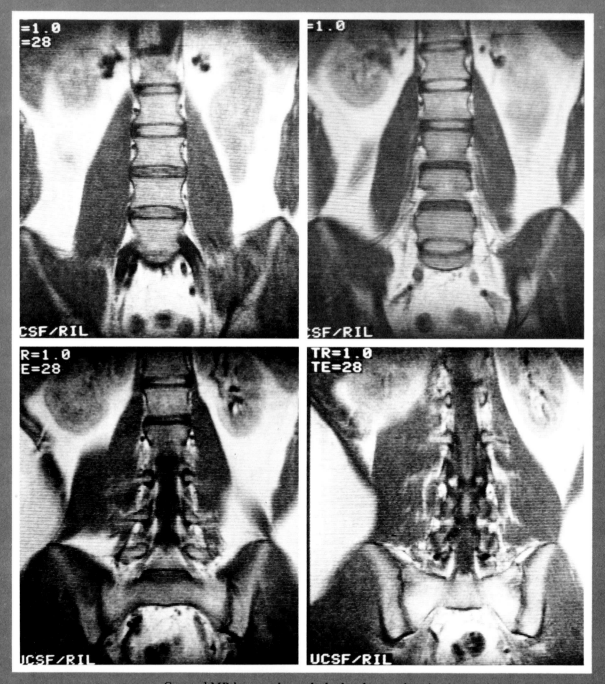

Coronal MR images through the lumbosacral region in an adult male (see Chapter 12)

Correlative Neuroanatomy of Computed Tomography and Magnetic Resonance Imaging

J. de GROOT, M.D., Ph.D.
Professor of Anatomy and Radiology
University of California, San Francisco

With contributions on Magnetic Resonance Imaging
CATHERINE M. MILLS, M.D.
Assistant Professor of Radiology
University of California, San Francisco

Line Drawings by
L. LYONS, M.A.
Medical Illustrator, Ventura, California

LEA & FEBIGER PHILADELPHIA
1984

LEA & FEBIGER
600 Washington Square
Philadelphia, Pa. 19106
U.S.A.
(215)922-1330

Library of Congress Cataloging in Publication Data

De Groot, J.
    Correlative neuroanatomy of computed tomography and
magnetic resonance imaging.

    Bibliography: p.
    Includes index.
    1. Central nervous system—Diseases—Diagnosis.
2. Central nervous system—Radiography.   3. Tomography.
4. Nuclear magnetic resonance—Diagnostic use.
I. Title.   [DNLM: 1. Nervous system—Radiography.
2. Nuclear magnetic resonance.   3. Tomography, X-ray
computed.   WL 141 D321c]
RC361.D424   1984   616.8'097572   83-22175
ISBN 0-8121-0917-1

PRINTED IN THE UNITED STATES OF AMERICA

Print Number: 5   4   3   2   1

Foreword

It is a genuine pleasure to introduce this book. I have had the good fortune to work with Jack De Groot first at the National Hospital in London and then on his home ground in San Francisco, and to benefit from both his enthusiasm for his subject and his magnanimity in communicating it. Like radiologists, anatomists are concerned primarily with morphology, but there is in both disciplines the temptation to schematise things, and present them other than as they really are. Dr. De Groot's interest is in the nervous system and its relationship to the structures around it, not in some idealised way, but as we may readily perceive it once we know how to look. This is evident in his perfection of a technique for the production of very fine slices of the entire head in different planes, demonstrating exquisitely the intimate juxtaposition of structures which are quite distinct in functional terms. The reader will also admire Dr. De Groot's ingenious dissections, which display the parts of interest with great clarity, but produce minimal disruption of their surroundings. While these methods combine to provide the tyro with a different, more faithful view of classical anatomy, they are equally instructive for those with wider experience in the neurosciences: as Pope said of Dr. Johnson, "New things are made familiar and familiar things are made new."

The introduction of computed tomography and the application of magnetic resonance to imaging have redirected the thrust of radiologic neuroanatomy, which previously bore only a passing resemblance to classical regional teaching, with the result that radiologists and anatomists hardly spoke the same language. Now the form and internal structure of the brain are there for all to see, and the first-year medical student can appreciate them almost as easily as the seasoned practitioner.

One of the merits of this book is the way in which images in various axial planes are mingled with those in the coronal and sagittal planes while all are related to a three dimensional vision. Although we may be able to construct abstract concepts of neuro-anatomy, they are often best expressed graphically, and the love of demonstrative images is another point of similarity between the radiologist and the anatomist.

I have suggested that the book you are about to read can be enjoyed on various planes. In this respect it resembles the work of Lewis Carroll. Although Carroll, as Charles Dodgson, was a mathematical logician, not an anatomist, he shared with Jack De Groot a keen interest in photography. His books, like this one, also have a strong graphic element: "'What is the use,' thought Alice, 'of a book without pictures or conversations?'" Pictures can be found here in abundance, and for those who enjoy conversation, it too is provided, in the form of the self-instructive catechisms that follow the text.

Ivory tower anatomy is of little practical value. I trust that the author of this textbook will not object too strongly to that statement—his frequent visits, have not only brightened the dark rooms of the radiology department, but also have kept him abreast of modern imaging procedures, enabling him to maintain a keen awareness of their practical applications. The fruit of the first of these applications, and something which gives me particular pleasure, is the collaboration with Cathy Mills, one of the first experts in clinical magnetic resonance imaging. The second, the introduction into the text of selected examples of pathology, illustrates effectively *why* clinicians need to be familiar with the way in which their patients are put together.

IVAN MOSELEY

National Hospital, London

Preface

A decade has passed since a new approach to brain imaging was introduced by Sir Godfrey N. Hounsfield and Allan M. Cormack. The method, *computed tomography (CT),* has now become widely accepted as the primary radiologic diagnostic procedure. Worldwide recognition of the method's importance and impact occurred in 1979, when the Nobel Prize in Physiology and Medicine was awarded to Sir Hounsfield and Dr. Cormack.

Another promising new method has become available that uses the principles of *nuclear magnetic resonance (NMR or MR)* to provide images of normal and abnormal human structures and indicate their chemical composition. The underlying basic, normal neuroanatomy, of course, remains the same as that used in computed tomography of the head and spine.

It is not surprising that in the last few years several atlases have appeared as reference works for the sectional, tomographic anatomy of CT or MR. It is remarkable, however, that no basic text is available for the teaching of CT or MR anatomy that systematically uses three-dimensional concepts that combine normal, gross neuroanatomic illustrations with the CT and MR images of normal subjects and of patients with lesions in the brain or spine.

This manual is intended to provide medical students, interns, and residents with a simple means to compare the main structures of the normal brain, skull, and spine with corresponding computer tomograms and MR images. A second goal is to refer the location of these structures and spaces within the brain and spine to major intracranial or spinal landmarks, so that the reader can put the *level of each section* or tomogram in perspective. Drawings, photographs, and radiologic images are thus used to instill an understanding of the three-dimensional nature of the brain and spine. Examples of changes seen in certain *clinical conditions* and self-testing questions and cases give an added dimension to the book by providing immediate feedback.

San Francisco, California   J. DE GROOT

Acknowledgments

Many friends and colleagues, here and abroad, have been most gracious by sharing their knowledge with us, by teaching understanding, or by allowing their illustrations to be used.

Sincerest thanks are due to Hans Newton, M.D., and David Norman, M.D., of the Department of Radiology, University of California, San Francisco. Their warm encouragement was matched by their splendid teaching file, from which several illustrations in this book stem.

The MR illustrations were most graciously provided and discussed by Catherine Mills, M.D., Radiologic Imaging Laboratory, University of California, San Francisco (Director; Leon Kaufman, Ph.D.). The generosity of Alan Goldfien, M.D., Director of the Health Careers Opportunity Grant, University of California, San Francisco, is acknowledged with appreciation; the production of many illustrations depended on this funding.

Messrs. J.D. Ritchey and D.R. Akers were most helpful in preparing and photographing many of the anatomic specimens.

Ms. Alana Schilling skillfully and repeatedly typed much of the manuscript.

The photographs used in Figures 3.3, 4.3, 6.11, 7.9A, 8.4A, 9.2, and 9.9 are derived from *Computer Reformations of the Brain and Skull Base* by Unsöld, Ostertag, De Groot, and Newton (Heidelberg, Springer Verlag, 1982). The illustrations used in Figures 11.14, 12.13, and 12.14 originally appeared in *Computed Tomography in the Evaluation of Trauma* edited by M.P. Federle and M. Brant-Zawadski (Baltimore, Williams and Wilkins, 1982). General Electric, Medical Systems, graciously provided Figures 7.4, 7.9B, and 10.5C. The permission to use these illustrations is gratefully acknowledged.

The cordial cooperation of the designer, Howard King and the publisher's staff, especially Thomas Colaiezzi, is sincerely appreciated. Last, but not least: my wife assisted in all aspects of the work; without her the book would not have been completed.

J. de G.

Contents

Correlative Neuroanatomy
of Computed Tomography
and Magnetic Resonance
Imaging

1. General Introduction

Computed tomography (CT) and *magnetic resonance (MR) imaging* are methods developed in the last decade that result in the visualization of detailed cross-sectional anatomy of portions of the human body. Studies of the normal neurocranium and its contents and of the vertebral column and the contents of the vertebral canal are of particular interest to clinical neurologists and neurosurgeons. Pathologic anatomy in numerous forms may be readily demonstrated, such as abnormal calcifications, brain edema, hydrocephalus, many types of tumors and cysts, hemorrhages, large aneurysms, and vascular malformations. Not surprisingly, therefore, the following statement was made in 1977: "It is now beyond question that CT is the primary neurodiagnostic procedure; it has largely replaced angiography, air studies, and isotope scanning" (T.H. Newton, University of California at San Francisco).

Computed tomography scanning, besides being "noninterventional," fast, and rather safe, has a high degree of sensitivity. Its specificity, however, is relatively limited. Therefore, in the presence of an abnormality, *correlation with clinical history and physical examination* is an absolute requirement for making a tentative neuropathologic diagnosis from a series of scans. Such a correlation is similarly important when using MR. Angiography or the injection of a contrast solution (with CT only) may be necessary to define and characterize a lesion.

The most modern imaging method, MR, is still in the developmental stage in terms of speed and general use. It promises, however, to be a safe method by which aspects of function and chemical tissue composition can be determined, thus giving added dimensions to an anatomic analysis. As with the CT method, correlation with a careful history and a thorough physical examination is important for the interpretation of the MR image.

Computed Tomography: Technical Comments

The CT scanning apparatus rotates a narrow x-ray beam around the head or spine. The amount of x rays transmitted is quantitated by detectors on the opposite side of the body. The quantity of x rays absorbed in small volumes of brain is computed by means of a series of simultaneous equations or an "algorithm." In most cases absorption is proportional to the density of the tissue. Each volume unit (measuring, e.g., 0.5 mm square by 1.5 mm in depth) is given a numerical *density value,* which by means of a digital-analog converter is translated to a pictorial element (pixel) on a *gray scale* (see Chapter 2). Images composed of many black, white, and gray pixels represent slices through skull or spine, meninges, brain, cord, vessels, or other tissues. The thickness of CT slices can be set in most modern scanners to vary from 10 mm to 1.5 mm. (The images in this book were obtained with a GE 8800 scanner.) In CT images, black represents low-density structures (with little attenuation of the x-ray beam), and white represents high-density structures (with much attenuation). The range of numerical attenuation values that the gray scale represents can be varied; a setting at which brain tissue is visualized to better advantage is commonly used. Sometimes bone needs to be examined in great detail (e.g., when fractures are suspected); occasionally soft tissues require additional settings. The gray scale in MR images has a different meaning (see Chapter 2).

Tissue density can change pathologically: hyperemia or freshly clotted hemorrhage appears more dense and edema, less dense, in CT images. The diagnostic sensitivity of CT scanning is increased by the use of iodinated contrast agents injected intravenously. These agents often pass into abnormal tissues through defects in the blood-brain barrier. Iodine in the contrast agent absorbs a large quantity of x rays, thus making the lesion more visible. Contrast in MR images depends on different *tissue properties,* such as the so-called T1 and T2 relaxation times, the hydrogen density, and the resonant motion of hydrogen protons in a magnetic field.

Magnetic Resonance Imaging: Technical Comments

A new, highly promising modality in neuroradiology is MR imaging. The MR imager used for this book (Diasonics) includes a 3.5 kilogauss superconducting magnet and saddle-shaped imaging coils (Fig. 1.1). The gradient coils modifying the main magnetic field do not exceed 1 gauss/cm, with a rise time of 1 msec. These gradients are essential in the spatial encoding of the MR image. Shielding from external radiofrequency sources is provided by enclosing the magnet and patient bed in copper mesh.

Nuclei with an odd number of protons, neutrons, or both are like magnets in a strong magnetic field. *Hydrogen* is currently the focus of MR imaging technology, as it is the most ubiquitous of the body's elements with this requisite nuclear configuration. In a magnetic field the previously randomly positioned protons become aligned in a parallel or antiparallel direction. This alignment produces a net magnetic moment, or *vector*, in the direction of the main magnetic field. The energy state of the protons is raised, and the net magnetic vector is shifted by the application of a *radiofrequency pulse* specific for hydrogen in a given magnetic field strength. The amplitude and duration of the radiofrequency pulse determines the change in the direction of the net magnetic vector. *The protons excited by a radiofrequency pulse emit energy as a radiofrequency signal as they return to their equilibrium state.* The ap-

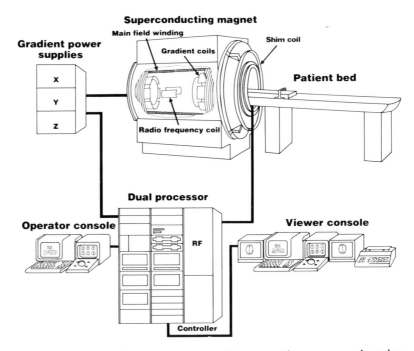

FIG. 1.1. Illustration of components used in magnetic resonance imaging.

plication of gradients to the main magnetic field produces spatial encoding of the protons, since each proton emits a radiofrequency signal that corresponds to a specific position in the gradient field.

The imaging techniques used in this book are the *spin echo* and *inversion recovery* sequences. The instrument parameters, which are varied to produce tissue contrast with the spin echo technique, are the *pulse sequence interval* and the *echo delay*. The *pulse sequence interval*, or *repetition time (TR)*, is the time interval between repeated radiofrequency perturbations of a volume in the sample. The *echo delay*, or *echo time (TE)*, is the time between radiofrequency excitation of the nuclei and the receipt of a signal or *spin echo* from the nuclei. The pulse sequence intervals most often used are 0.5, 1.0, 1.5, and 2.0 secs. The echo delays are 28 and 56 msec. Inversion recovery sequences are usually performed with a pulse interval of 1.0 sec. and an inversion time (TI) of 0.4 sec.

T1   The alignment of protons after placement in a magnetic field occurs exponentially, described by the *time constant T1*. It is also the time constant for *return to equilibrium (relaxation)* following a radiofrequency disturbance. This return to equilibrium necessitates an energy exchange between the nucleus and the magnetic moments of the surrounding tissue elements, the *lattice*. This energy exchange *can only occur at the resonant frequency;* consequently, the vibrational state of the molecules in the lattice affects the rate of exchange. Molecules within the lattice structure are not immobile; rather, they have vibrational frequencies with distributions that depend on size, temperature, binding, etc. The range of vibrational frequencies of small molecules, such as water, is wide, covering many frequencies in addition to the resonant frequency, and resulting in only a small amount of energy for exchange and, consequently, a long relaxation time.

The vibration frequency range of larger molecules is lower; therefore, the relaxation process is more efficient. Physical characteristics of the sample such as temperature, viscosity, and molecular structure of solutes all affect T1. These factors normally result in a *long T1 for solids and "pure" liquids* (such as water or cerebrospinal fluid [CSF]) and a *short T1 for impure liquids* (containing large molecules, such as blood in an extravasation or hemorrhage). The T1 relaxation time is also called the spin-lattice or thermal relaxation time (another term, longitudinal relaxation time).

Differences in tissue contrast due to T1 are selectively enhanced by *alterations in the interval between repetitive radiofrequency perturbations* of the sample. *Tissues with a short T1 (rapid magnetization) produce relatively a greater signal compared to tissues with a longer T1 (longer magnetization) if the pulse interval is short.*

INVERSION RECOVERY

The *inversion recovery technique* of signal acquisition also introduces T1 dependence in the MR image. In this technique, the net magnetization vector is first inverted and then allowed to recover for a time, TI. The recovery interval can be manipulated to permit tissues with long T1 relaxation values to be observed at times when their signal is nearly zero, while tissues with shorter T1 values yield considerable signal. *Inversion recovery images produce exquisite differentiation between gray and white matter* due to the short T1 of the latter. However, the contrast between various tissues with long T1 relaxation times is decreased, limiting their differentiation, and therefore their clinical applicability.

T2

The T2, or transverse relaxation time, is the exponential constant that characterizes the decay of the signal intensity from perturbed tissue; it reflects the proton's loss of coherent resonance after a radiofrequency pulse. The inhomogeneities in the internal magnetic field of the sample alter the resonant frequencies of the individual nuclei, resulting in the extinction of the resonance signal by loss of coherence. *Solids* have static internal magnetic fields causing strong variations in the local magnetic fields and a corresponding *short T2;* thus the *decay of their signal is rapid. Liquids* have rapid molecular motion, which decreases the effects of internal magnetic fields and increases the time in which nuclei resonate coherently, or in phase, resulting in a *long T2.* The T2 characterizes energy exchanges between nuclear spins of the same type and is therefore also called the *spin-spin relaxation time.*

The effects on the image of T2 variations between tissues may be selectively enhanced by varying the *echo time. If the echo time is increased, the signal intensity from tissues with long relaxation times will be maintained relative to tissues with shorter T2 in which the loss of coherence is rapid.*

Procedures and Planes

A series of 10 to 15 scans (sections or "cuts"), each representing a 10-mm-thick slice, is usually required for a complete study of the brain. With the most modern CT apparatus each scan takes only a few seconds. Thinner sections (1.5 mm in width) can be obtained if better spatial resolution is needed (see section in Chapter 3 on volume-averaging). Thin sections are required for the "reformation" of images of good quality (see Chapter 7). Most MR images in this book represent a 7-mm thick section; the distance between the centers of two contiguous sections is 11 mm.

From the starting level, which is usually at the foramen magnum upwards, a series of brain sections is taken by moving the table on which the patient is lying (normally in supine position) between scans, so that the last scan is taken through the top of the head (Fig. 1.2). Images through the spine are started at the lowest level of a series, at right angles to the axis of the spinal column. Each image, whether obtained by the CT or by the MR imaging method, is viewed as if standing at the feet of the patient: the left side of the image is the patient's right side, unless marked differently.

At first, in 1973, the normal examination with CT was performed with the head tilted up, at 15° to 20° to the orbito-meatal plane (a plane through the lateral edge of both orbits and the external auditory meatus on both sides). This head position was associated with the use of a waterbag around the back of the head.

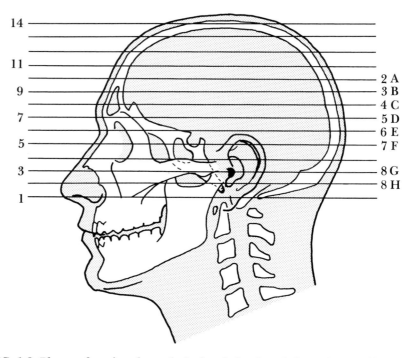

FIG. 1.2. Planes of section through the head. Sections 1 through 12 indicate the sequence of routine scanning (1, at the level of the foramen magnum; 4, at the infraorbitomeatal level). The chapters discussing slices A through H are indicated on the right.

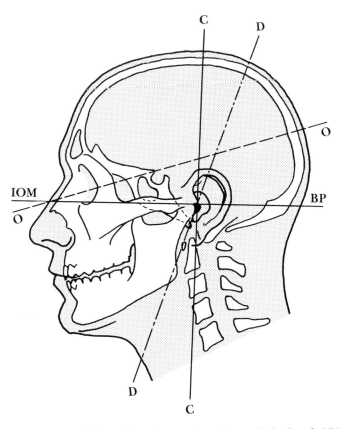

FIG. 1.3. Normally used base plane for sections through the head. IOM-BP-Infraorbitomeatal base plane; O-O-orbital axis; C-C-true coronal plane; D-D-coronal plane used in direct computed tomography.

More recently, the orientation of routine head scans is parallel to the *infraorbitomeatal base plane* (Fig. 1.3). This position results in horizontal, or axial, images. As the patient can easily be moved within the scanner, a lower level at the foramen magnum is the usual starting level for a complete series of scans through the brain.

Computer "reformations" from a series of thin sections allow visualization in any desired plane (e.g., the midsagittal plane) anywhere in the head (see Chapter 7). *Coronal sections* are often extremely useful for the visualization of structures lying at the base of the brain, in the high convexity area, and close to the incisura of the tentorium; the slope of the tentorium itself is often better seen on a coronal section (see Chapter 7). Orbital structures are either scanned parallel to, or with negative angulation to, the infraorbitomeatal plane (Fig. 1.3). Detailed comparison between contents of the left and right orbit is preferably done in

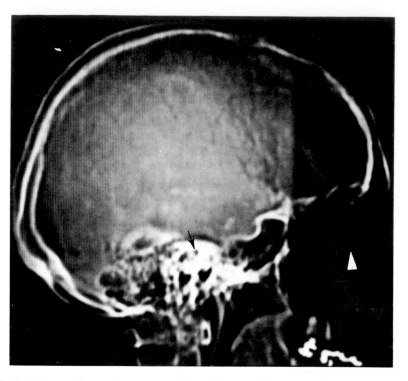

FIG. 1.4. Normal lateral scout view. Note the resemblance to a lateral plain skull film. The external auditory meatus *(arrow)* and the lower rim of the orbit *(arrowhead)* can be readily distinguished

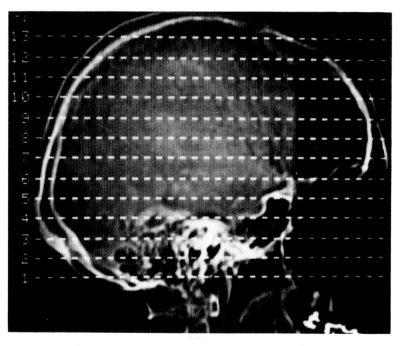

FIG. 1.5. Normal lateral scout view, with planes of computed tomographic cuts indicated *(broken lines)*. Note that the first cut is at the level of the foramen magnum; the last cut is close to the top of the head.

planes at right angles to each *orbital axis* (see Chapter 9). The MR imaging method permits sections to be made directly in any plane. The position of the head or spine, the orientation of the plane used, and the level of each section can be documented by means of "scout views" (digital radiographs made with the CT scanner, comparable to plain skull or spine films; see Figs. 1.4 and 1.5).

In this book, a high section (not the topmost one) is discussed first for the purpose of easy introduction to the relatively simple anatomic analysis of CT and MR images at that level. Successively lower scans are then taken up in the following chapters. Images through the orbit are reviewed in Chapter 9. Chapter 10 contains comments on the region of the craniovertebral junction, while a discussion of the spine and spinal cord is found in Chapters 11 and 12.

2. Lateral Ventricle
(Anatomic Slice A)

Normal Anatomy

The main structures and spaces seen in this high slice or "cut" are the scalp, skull cap, cortex, with sulci and gyri; white matter (here sometimes called centrum semiovale); falx cerebri (dura); subarachnoid space containing CSF, and lateral ventricles (containing CSF), all within a background of air (Fig. 2.1). Most of these structures are found in several other slices, both higher and lower ones. It is therefore of considerable importance not only to recognize at each level the main structures and spaces themselves, but also to put them in perspective: What lies higher? What is found lower? Which portion of the entire structure is seen at this particular level?

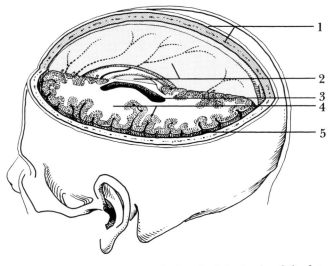

FIG. 2.1. Drawing of an axial slice at the level of the body of the lateral ventricle. *1,* Scalp, skull cap (calvaria); *2,* corpus callosum, falx; *3,* lateral ventricle, superior sagittal sinus; *4,* centrum semiovale, cerebral cortex; *5,* subarachnoid space.

13

The *falx* (cerebri) and its lower, tent-shaped, flared continuation, the *tentorium* (cerebelli), will be encountered in many CT sections through the head (Fig. 2.2); a sure understanding of how each section (anatomic, CT, or MR) is cut with respect to these dura folds is most helpful in localizing levels, compartments, and regions. Similarly, the *ventricular system* has a characteristic shape and configuration (Fig. 2.3); its typical cross sections are excellent references, at each level, to determine localization within the brain (Fig. 2.4).

The combination of dural folds, ventricular system, and midsagittal brain structures above or below the tentorium provides an additional framework of reference (Figs. 2.5 and 2.6). A midsagittal section with the main arteries will be used to indicate the level of each section in this and subsequent chapters (Fig. 2.7).

On the anatomic slice A some of the same structures seen in Figure 2.1 are seen in a horizontal or axial plane (Fig. 2.8). The *skull cap* with its dura and *falx* is covered with *scalp* (slightly irregular in this series of anatomic sections because of widespread neurofibromatosis). The somewhat dilated *lateral ventricles* are separated by a thin *septum* and are flanked by the left and right caudate nuclei. Portions of the *corpus callosum* lie anterior and

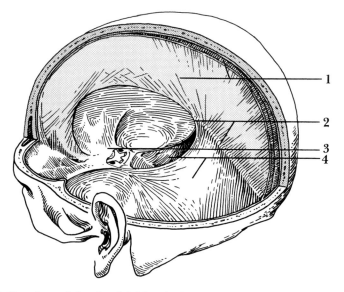

FIG. 2.2. Drawing of the dural folds within the cranial cavity. *1*, Falx (cerebri), superior sagittal sinus; *2*, apex of the tentorium and highest point of the seam between falx and tentorium, straight sinus; *3*, planum sphenoidale with anterior clinoid processes, free edge of the right half of the tentorium; *4*, incisura of the tentorium ("notch"), left half of the tentorium.

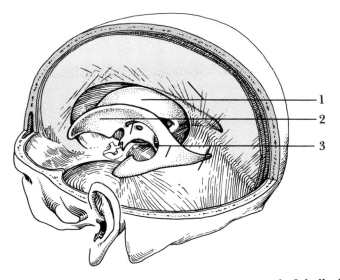

FIG. 2.3. Outline of the ventricular system on a background of skull with dura. *1*, Body of right lateral ventricle, falx; *2*, anterior (frontal) horn of left lateral ventricle, third ventricle (in midplane); *3*, aqueduct, atrium of left lateral ventricle, left half of the tentorium. Note the proximity of the inferior horns to the tentorium.

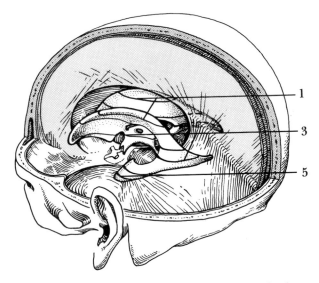

FIG. 2.4. Illustration of a "sliced" ventricular system on a background of skull with dura (fourth ventricle not shown). *1*, Highest level (Figs. 2.1 and 2.3; see Chapter 2); *3*, level through mid-third ventricle and atria (Figs. 4.1 and 4.3; see Chapter 4); *5*, level through the lower hypothalamus and inferior horn (Figs. 6.1 and 6.4; see Chapter 6).

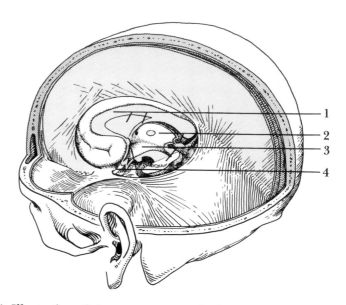

FIG. 2.5. Illustration of the structures seen in the opening of the falx and the incisura. *1,* Corpus callosum, septum, fornix; *2,* thalamus, pineal gland; *3,* hypothalamus, left half of midbrain; *4,* left optic nerve, infundibular recess of third ventricle.

posterior to the ventricles in this section, as well as above these CSF-containing spaces.

A now firmly established convention is to view each slice of a series of sections as if standing at the feet of the supine patient; the left side of the anatomic photograph, CT image, or MR image thus represents the right side of the patient (unless indicated otherwise).

The lateral ventricles are situated below a bilateral region of *white matter:* the left and right *centrum semiovale.* The region just lateral to the caudate nucleus is sometimes referred to as *corona radiata;* this fiber bundle continues in lower sections as internal capsule. The cerebral *cortical ribbon* is clearly seen; it is separated from the dura by the *subarachnoid space.*

In Figure 2.8, a difference in cortical thickness is seen on either side of the central sulcus (precentral gyrus is thicker), so that the *frontal lobes* can be distinguished from the *parietal lobes.* On a CT or MR scan this differentiation is seldom possible with precision.

Figure 2.9 is a normal, axial MR image showing the same structures as described in Figures 2.1 and 2.8. The skull is black (no signal), the *scalp* white (high signal) and the *temporalis muscle* is gray (intermediate signal). The *ventricles* and *caudate nuclei* are

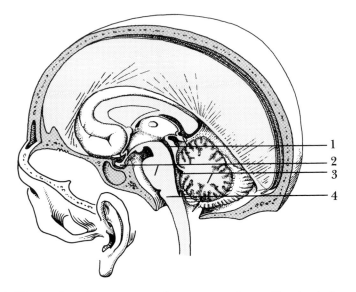

FIG. 2.6. Illustration of structures and spaces seen in a midsagittal plane. *1*, Aqueduct, quadrigeminal plate (tectum), pineal gland; *2*, pituitary gland within sella turcica, pons; *3*, fourth ventricle, cerebellum; *4*, medulla, foramen magnum.

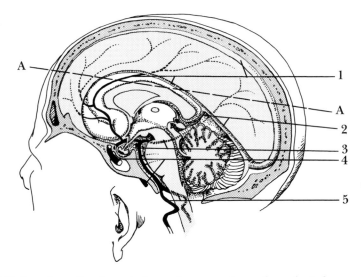

FIG. 2.7. Drawing of major arteries and venous channels projected on a midsagittal plane. The level of slice A is indicated by line A-A. *1*, Branches of anterior cerebral artery, inferior and superior sagittal sinuses; *2*, great cerebral vein (of Galen), straight sinus; *3*, basilar artery, right posterior cerebral artery coursing behind the brain stem; *4*, internal carotid arteries; *5*, vertebral arteries. (Right posterior communicating artery shown behind infundibulum).

clearly seen in this spin echo image; the *cortical ribbon* is whiter than the grayish *centrum semiovale*. The *falx* is represented by a thin black line; the *blood* within its venous channels is black (no signal), provided it is flowing freely and does not contain turbulences. Stagnant or turbulent blood has a high or intermediate signal (see Fig. 6.7). The air around the head is shown as black.

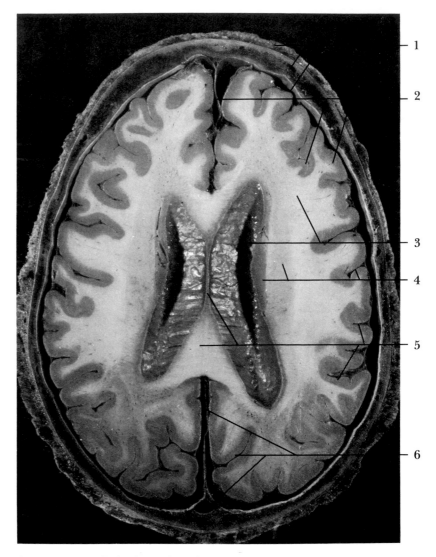

FIG. 2.8. Anatomic horizontal section at the level of the bodies of the lateral ventricles. *1*, Scalp, skull, subarachnoid space; *2*, falx in interhemispheric fissure, frontal lobe gyri; *3*, body of left lateral ventricle, centrum semiovale; *4*, caudate nucleus, corona radiata, central sulcus; *5*, corpus callosum, septum, parietal lobe gyri; *6*, posterior falx, parieto-occipital fissure, superior sagittal sinus. Note that this brain has enlarged ventricles.

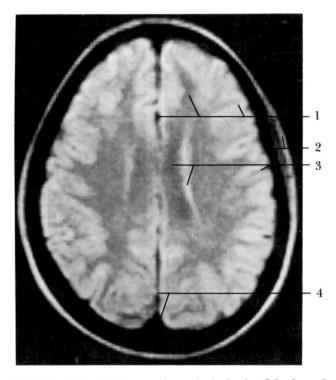

FIG. 2.9. Axial MR (spin echo) image through the body of the lateral ventricles. *1*, Vessel in interhemispheric fissure, white matter, cortex; *2*, temporalis muscle, scalp; *3*, lateral ventricle, caudate nucleus, central sulcus; *4*, posterior falx, superior sagittal sinus, skull.

Gray Scale Structures on CT images are usually depicted with such a "gray scale" (from white to black): black indicates no attenuation of the x-ray beam and therefore no absorption in a tissue, and little x-ray density; white means high density of a tissue, a high absorption level, and a high attenuation of the x-ray beam.

The contrast in an MR image is the result of the interaction of the images with the T1 and T2 relaxation times, the hydrogen density, and the state of motion of hydrogen. These images are substantially different from conventional x-ray radiographic and computed tomogram images, which are dependent on electron density. The factors contributing to the MR image contrast and their diagnostic implications are not completely understood. Nevertheless, the interactions of these factors with the imaging system yield high soft-tissue contrast, providing a wide range of intensities for tissues that were not previously well differentiated on the basis of their electron densities.

The gray scale in the MR images shows fat as the brightest tissue, followed by marrow and cancellous bone, brain and spinal cord, viscera, muscle, fluid-filled cavities, ligaments and tendons, rapidly flowing blood, compact bone, and air, in decreasing order of intensity. Tissues with high intensity on a spin echo image have a short T1 or a long T2, or both. Low-intensity areas result from a long T1 or a short T2, or both. Variations of the echo time and the repetition time discriminate between tissues as a function of the relative lengths of their relaxation times.

Computed Tomography Densities

Each of the tissues or fluids represented in a routine CT examination normally has a characteristic CT density that varies between black (lowest density) and white (highest density) on the viewing screen or photographic image (Fig. 2.10 and Table 2.1). The individual characteristic density can be seen best when the viewing window or "window width" is adjusted to include a small range of densities that are higher to lower than the structure examined. Since the difference in density between gray and white matter of

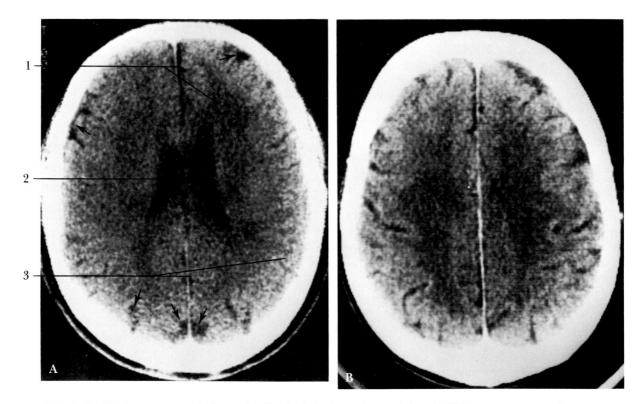

FIG. 2.10. CT images at and above the level of the lateral ventricles. A. Without contrast enhancement. *1*, Interhemispheric fissure with falx, centrum semiovale; *2*, body of left lateral ventricle, caudate nucleus; *3*, posterior falx, parietal cortex. There are some low-density areas in the cortex *(arrows)*: deep sulci or small infarcts, or both. B. With contrast enhancement (the next higher section). Note that the difference between gray and white areas is more pronounced, and the falx is easier to see; in general, the image is clearer.

TABLE 2.1. *CT Coefficients of Absorption in Hounsfield Units (HU)*

Air	−1000 HU	Edema	8 to 17 HU	Clotted Blood	40 to 80 HU
Fat	−80 HU	White Matter	24 to 36 HU	Glioma	9 to 60 to 800 HU
H_2O	0 HU	Gray Matter	32 to 50 HU	Calcification	80 to 1000 HU
CSF	0 to 16 HU	Flowing Blood	20 to 50 HU	Bone	up to 1000 HU

the brain is small (see Table 2.1), the scale is normally set so as to include both components.

Window Width   The window width is an expression of the set sensitivity of the gray scale in CT: a relatively narrow window permits differentiation between slightly different densities, whereas a very wide window setting distinguishes little between very dense (white on the viewing screen, e.g., bone) and non-dense (black on the viewing screen, e.g., air or CSF) (Fig. 2.11). A window width of 80 to 150 Hounsfield units is usually adopted for routine scans of brain structures. In Figures 2.10A and B, the skull is clearly seen as a dense (white) structure around the brain; details such as diploë or

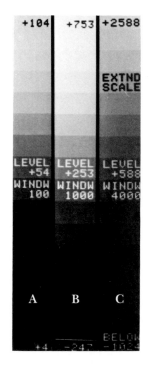

FIG. 2.11. Three different settings of window width: *a*, Normal setting for brain tissue; *b*, regular "bone window" setting; *c*, special setting for greater detail of bone structures.

sutures cannot be seen with the usual window width. The falx can rarely be seen clearly (unless partially calcified as may occur in normal older persons), nor is the scalp clearly seen in its entirety. Cerebrospinal fluid spaces and gray or white matter areas are easily distinguished.

Contrast Enhancement

The falx and other structures can be demonstrated quite well on contrast-enhanced scans (Figs. 2.10B and 2.12). "Contrast," a nonionized, iodine-containing solution (Hexabrix or Conray) is injected intravenously in an amount proportional to body weight. Such an injection causes the vessels to be more clearly seen, as well as all areas where there is no (or a deficient) blood-brain barrier: the falx and tentorium, tumors, necrotic areas, etc. The cortex, which is more vascular, now stands out more clearly from the white matter. The effect of such a contrast enhancement lasts

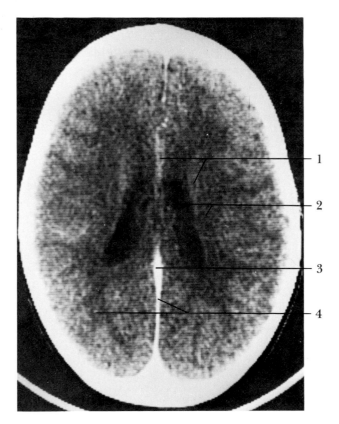

FIG. 2.12. CT section after contrast enhancement. The plane of section is higher anteriorly and lower posteriorly than in Figure 2.10A, so that the anterior part of the ventricles is not imaged. *1*, pericallosal arteries, caudate nucleus; *2*, body of left lateral ventricle, white matter; *3*, inferior sagittal sinus, and beginning of straight sinus; *4*, right optic radiation, posterior falx.

up to 2 hours in normal persons. This procedure is well tolerated in most patients, and the contrast material is readily excreted, but for those persons who have an iodine allergy the procedure is contraindicated.

The spaces around the brain containing CSF are usually not seen unless the subarachnoid space is abnormally wide; however, between the hemispheres and in large fissures the CSF density can be identified in most cases. The ventricular CSF has practically the same density as the subarachnoid space despite a slight difference in protein content. (See the ventricular system shown in Figs. 2.3 and 2.4). It is very important to recognize (and report) the size and configuration of the ventricles: Are they normal? dilated? symmetrical? displaced?

A comparable MR image through the lateral ventricles is shown in Figure 2.13. Note that the skull is seen in several areas as two black lines (cortical, "waterless" bone) on either side of a

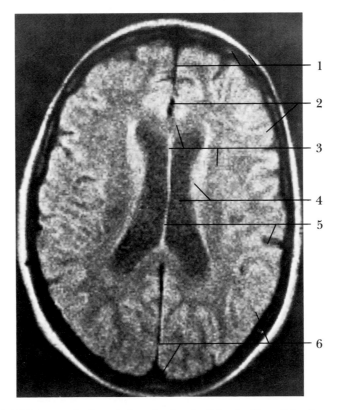

FIG. 2.13. MR image (spin echo) at the level of the bodies of the lateral ventricles (slightly dilated). *1*, Scalp, skull, falx; *2*, pericallosal arteries, cortex of frontal lobe; *3*, septum, genu of corpus callosum, corona radiata; *4*, left lateral ventricle, caudate nucleus; *5*, septum, sulcus with artery; *6*, posterior falx, superior sagittal sinus, parietal cortex.

gray zone (diploë or marrow, containing more mobile hydrogen protons). The gray and the white matter areas of the brain can be readily distinguished by this spin echo method of imaging.

Altered Anatomy

A CT image differing from a normal one is shown in Figure 2.14. What are the changes compared to Figures 2.10 and 2.12? There are several streak-artifacts, especially anteriorly and on the right side. These are caused by the sharp demarcations between very high and low densities ("overshoot" effect). The patient had several pathologic areas at lower levels (not shown).

Clinically abnormal images of a 60-year-old patient are seen in Figure 2.15, taken in the emergency room after trauma to the head. Note the "mass effect." How should the images be interpreted? The number of Hounsfield units of the parafalcian high density, measured by a special CT method, was 73, a number in the density range of freshly clotted blood. The patient apparently

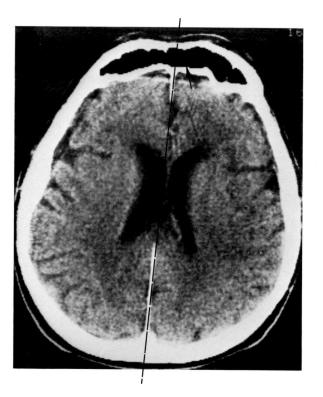

FIG. 2.14. CT image at the level of the lateral ventricles (image is lower anteriorly, higher posteriorly than Figure 2.10A). A large frontal air sinus *(arrow)* is present; the right lateral ventricle appears larger than the left one. There is a slight right to left mass effect across the (interrupted) midline. The head is slightly rotated sideways.

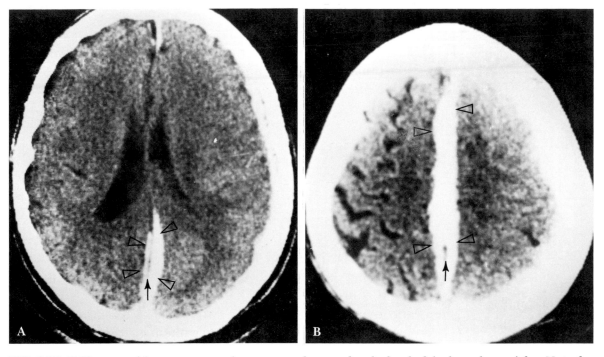

FIG. 2.15. CT images without contrast enhancement, above and at the level of the lateral ventricles. Note the linear area of high density *(arrowheads)* on both sides along the falx *(arrow)*. There is mass effect: A. The lateral ventricle is compressed. B. The cortical sulci are partially effaced on the right side (edema).

had bled from one or more torn superficial veins that drain into the superior sagittal sinus. Often such a hemorrhage is into the subdural space; in this case, the blood is clearly in the subdural space between the hemispheres.

Another example of the effect of a rapidly growing mass is seen in Figure 2.16A. A right to left shift is indicated by the bowing of the falx; the white matter contains an irregular area of lower density than normal. In Figure 2.16B, a similar low-density area is seen partially surrounding a mass (of a different patient). The low-density zone represents edema of the brain. It is a higher section than the one seen in Figure 2.16A. The masses in both cases represent metastatic tumor. Slow-growing, benign tumors may not have a surrounding rim of edema. Figure 2.17 represents an MR image of a 27-year-old patient in whom a tentative diagnosis of multiple sclerosis had been made. Computed tomography examinations made earlier, with and without contrast, did not show any abnormality, at least not conclusively. The white, patchy areas of Figure 2.17 probably indicate a change in the hydrogen or water content of the white matter, suggesting demyelination and confirming the diagnosis.

Before proceeding, review all the numbered structures in Figure 2.9. These structures have been discussed in the preceding pages. Now try to solve the clinical problems, then answer the questions; the case discussions are found in Chapter 13, and the answers to questions, in Chapter 14.

Clinical Cases (Glossary of clinical terms and abbreviations can be found on page 231)

CASE 1 A 58-year-old, single, white woman had been reasonably well until approximately 5 years earlier, when her friends noted gradual behavioral changes and decreased mental ability. She became unable to carry out complex tasks, and she was depressed and sometimes confused. Later she began to complain of forgetfulness and inability to "find the right words." Currently she had been admitted to the hospital for treatment of severe bronchopneumonia.

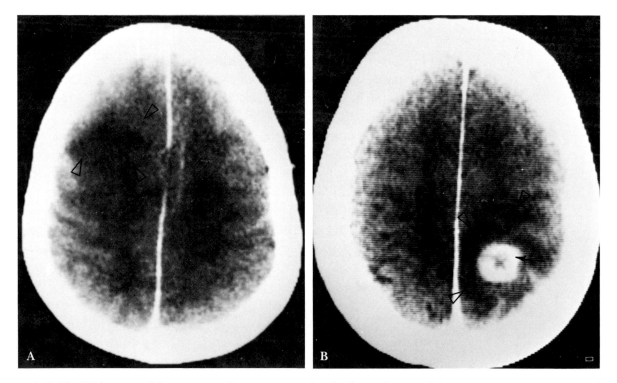

FIG. 2.16. CT images with contrast enhancement, at levels above the ventricles. A. Note the asymmetrical low-density area *(arrowheads)* and the slight displacement of midline. B. High in the brain of another patient, a high-density area with a low (necrotic?) center *(arrow)* is seen with surrounding low density *(arrowheads)*.

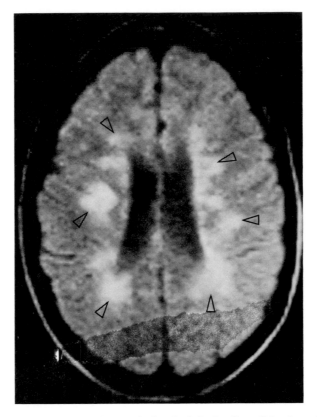

FIG. 2.17. MR image (spin echo) at the level of the bodies of the lateral ventricle. There are many patchy, high-signal intensity areas *(arrowheads)* around both ventricles; these represent demyelinated plaques, containing relatively more fluid with a long T2.

GPE: A thin, listless woman with senile changes in skin, cornea, and lens; peripheral mild arteriosclerosis. S/S of left-sided bronchopneumonia, with moderate fever. BP 125/80.

NEX: Marked confusion, disorientation X2; memory defects, especially for recent events. Difficulty of comprehension of speech; anomia. Generalized muscular weakness and atrophy; inability to wash and dress herself.

Lab Data: Unremarkable, except for WBC of 16,500.

CT Scan (Figs. 2.18A and B): Where is the neuropathologic process located anatomically? Are the ventricles normal in size (compare with a normal scan, Fig. 2.10)? What is your DDX? What other information would you require to make a definitive DX?

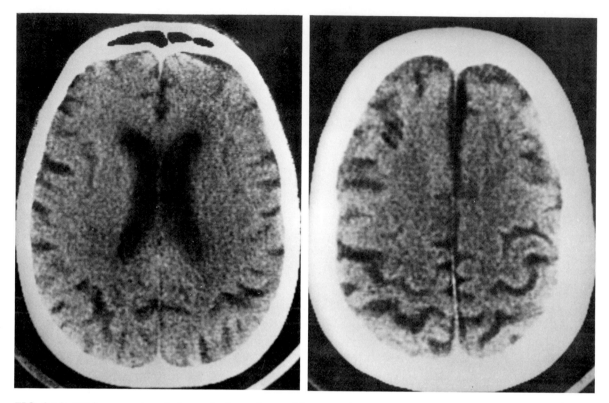

FIG. 2.18. CT images at and above the lateral ventricles. A. The ventricles appear dilated, and the sulci are clearly visible. B. The sulci and fissures are shown wider than normally seen at this age.

(Discussion of Case 1 on p. 195)

CASE 2

A 60-year-old, white, right-handed woman was admitted for observation after she had had a brief, convulsive episode (seizure). In the two-year period PTA, visiting relatives had noted a change in personality; she had become apathetic, and showed "silly" behavior, sometimes incoherence. Three months ago, a change in facial expression was noted ("flatness" of the left face); a few weeks ago a decreased swing of the left arm was noticed.

NEX: Oriented X3; marked loss of motor coordination; delayed recall 2/5 objects; inappropriate joking. L central facial weakness; weakness of LUE and LLE. DTR: increased L; L. Babinski's sign.

CT Scan (Figs. 2.19A and B): Which other test procedures would you think necessary? Where is the lesion? What is your DDX at this point?

Patient became rapidly worse, complained of headache, nausea, and poor eyesight; she then had two seizures. The neurosurgeons operated on her almost immediately. What do you expect they found? Why did the patient deteriorate so rapidly preoperatively?

(Discussion of Case 2 and additional illustrations on p. 196)

Questions

2a. What is the CT density (in Hounsfield Units) of bone? Of CSF?

2b. What has a higher CT density, gray matter or white matter?

2c. How can a sharply outlined and detailed CT image of a skull slice be obtained?

2d. How can the visibility of the falx on CT images be improved?

2e. Are the different densities of gray and white matter in the brain seen in MR images representing the same structures as in CT sections (compare Figs. 2.9 and 2.13 with Figs. 2.10 and 2.12)?

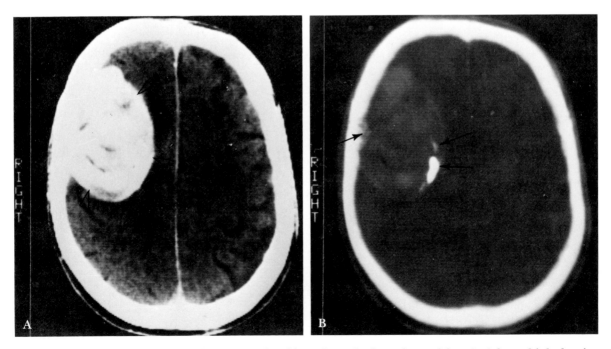

FIG. 2.19. Contrast-enhanced CT images at a level just above the lateral ventricles. A. A large high-density mass in the right frontal lobe *(arrowheads)* is seen; there is little mass effect. B. A "bone window" image is seen demonstrating the areas of calcium within the abnormal mass *(arrows)*.

2f. Why is the cortex more easily differentiated from white matter in contrast-enhanced CT scans?

2g. Define the infraorbitomeatal base plane.

2h. Does the tip of the anterior (frontal) horn of the lateral ventricle lie in a higher plane (parallel to the infraorbitomeatal base plane) than the interventricular foramen (of Monro)?

2i. In a routine series of CT scans, where is the first cut through the patient's head taken? Where is the last cut, ideally? Why?

2j. How can one accurately define (in an anatomic slice) the boundary between frontal and parietal lobe?

2k. How can one indicate, on CT scans, those structures that do not possess a blood-brain barrier? Why is that important?

3. Corpus Callosum; Lateral Ventricle (*Anatomic Slice B*)

Normal Anatomy

In the next lower slice the same structures as before are seen; however, additional portions of the ventricular system and the corpus callosum are shown in their characteristic shapes, positions, and CT densities.

The *body of the corpus callosum* was already present in slice A, but not emphasized (Fig. 2.8). It is a myelinated, low-density structure that extends between and above the bodies of the lateral ventricles, and blends with the white matter of thc *centrum semiovale* (Fig. 3.1). The *genu* of the corpus callosum lies anterior to the *anterior* (or frontal) *horns* of the lateral ventricles (Figs. 3.2 and

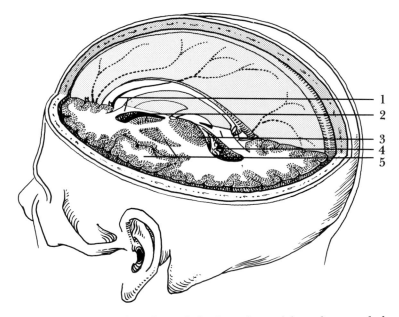

FIG. 3.1. Drawing of level B, through the lateral ventricle and upper thalamus. *1,* Pericallosal artery (branch of anterior cerebral artery), genu of corpus callosum; *2,* anterior (frontal) horn, caudate nucleus; *3,* thalamus, splenium of corpus callosum, great cerebral vein (of Galen); *4,* atrium with choroid plexus; *5,* upper temporal lobe, lateral (Sylvian) fissure and insula, putamen.

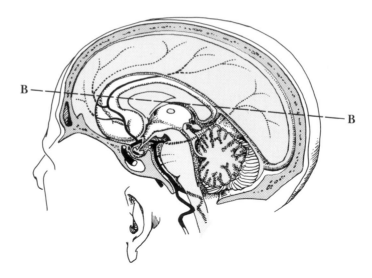

FIG. 3.2. Drawing of midsagittal structures and spaces to illustrate level of slice B.

3.3). The *splenium* is found between the widest portions of the ventricles and the *atria* (or trigones) with their extensive *choroid plexus.* The genu and splenium, together with the body of the corpus callosum, form a massive commissure between the two cerebral hemispheres. The relationship between *thalamus, caudate nucleus, putamen,* and *internal capsule,* although visible here and in Figure 3.3, will be discussed in Chapter 4.

The *lateral ventricles* have just begun to separate into their divisions: *body,* (top of the) *anterior* or frontal *horn, atrium* or trigone (Fig. 3.4). Review the ventricular system (Fig. 2.3). The lateral ventricles depicted in Figure 3.3 are dilated, a condition often found in old persons. The *frontal horns,* separated by the *septum,* lie behind the *genu* of the corpus callosum. Three gray masses, the *caudate nucleus, putamen,* and *thalamus,* are found between the frontal horn and atrium on each side at this level; the corona radiata has converged into an important fiber bundle, the *internal capsule,* lying between these gray masses (see Fig. 4.6).

The *temporal lobes* have made their appearance in Figure 3.3, as well as the *insulae* on the medial side of each *lateral fissure* with their branches of the *middle cerebral artery.* Just anterior to the genu course the *pericallosal arteries,* branches of the *anterior cerebral artery.* Just behind the splenium the *great cerebral vein* is about to drain into the *straight sinus,* which at a lower level forms a confluence with the *superior sagittal sinus* and a small occipital sinus.

Computed tomography images at this level correspond closely to the underlying anatomy (Figs. 3.5 and 3.6). The *genu* and *splenium* of the corpus callosum are identifiable. The configuration of the internal capsule between masses of gray *(thalamus, putamen,* and *caudate)* may vary between sections at slightly differ-

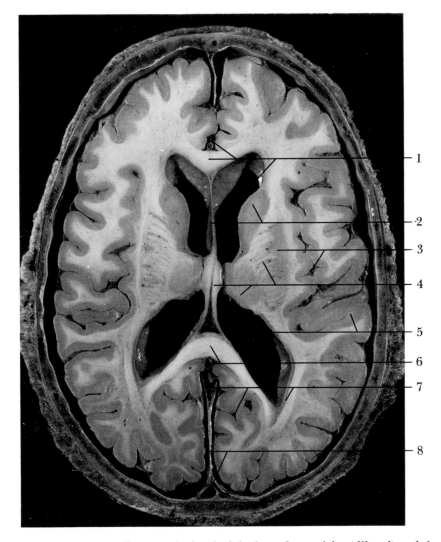

FIG. 3.3. Anatomic slice B at the level of the lateral ventricles (dilated) and the upper thalamus. *1,* Pericallosal arteries, genu of corpus callosum, left anterior (frontal horn); *2,* septum, head of caudate nucleus; *3,* upper portion of lentiform nucleus, lateral fissure; *4,* fornix, upper thalamus, internal capsule; *5,* (enlarged) atrium (choroid plexus lost in sectioning process), parietal gyri; *6,* great cerebral vein, splenium of corpus callosum; *7,* straight sinus, parieto-occipital fissure, left optic radiation; *8,* posterior falx, superior sagittal sinus. (Unsöld, R., Ostertag, C. B., De Groot J., and Newton, T. J.: Computer Reformations of the Brain and Skull Base. Berlin, Heidelberg, New York, Springer-Verlag, 1982.)

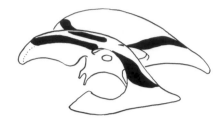

FIG. 3.4. Drawing of ventricular "slice" at the level of Figure 3.3.

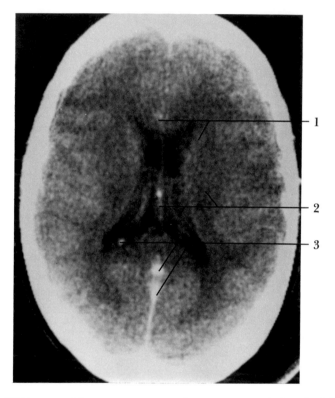

FIG. 3.5. CT image with some contrast enhancement at the level of the upper thalamus. *1*, Vessels anterior to genu of corpus callosum, anterior horn with head of caudate nucleus averaged-in, caudate nucleus; *2*, internal cerebral vein, choroid plexus in lateral ventricle, corona radiata; *3*, calcified portion of choroid plexus in atrium, calcium in pineal gland, straight sinus. Note asymmetry of frontal horns.

ent levels: these masses have just come into this picture, and "volume averaging" may affect their representation on a CT scan.

Volume Averaging

"Volume averaging" (sometimes referred to as "partial volume effect") results in a certain inaccuracy of imaging, especially in thick slices; if two or more structures are present within a given volume element (voxel), the resulting pixel (picture element) rep-

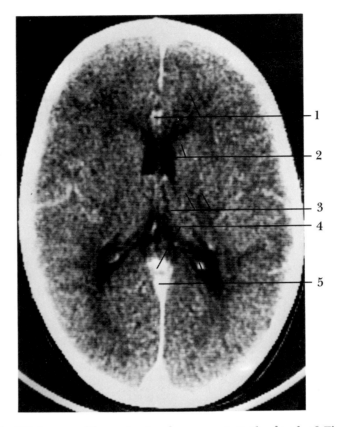

FIG. 3.6. CT image with contrast enhancement at the level of Figure 3.5. *1*, Pericallosal arteries, frontal white matter; *2*, septum, head of caudate nucleus; *3*, upper thalamus, internal capsule, putamen; *4*, internal cerebral veins averaged into splenium, calcified pineal gland; *5*, junction of great vein and straight sinus, slightly calcified choroid plexus.

resents a density that is the average of these structures (Figs. 3.7 and 3.8). This is most noticeable in volume elements where two or more very different densities are averaged, e.g., skull and subarachnoid space, or ventricle and brain tissue. In the first example, the very high density of the bone dominates the low density of the CSF, so that the high average density of the pixels at the transition zone make the skull look thicker in tangential cuts than it really is (Fig. 3.7). In the second example, the low CSF density and the density of brain, which is not so low, are averaged, thus diffusing the sharp boundary between ventricle and brain (Fig. 3.8). In thin, 1.5-mm-thick slices the density representation of each pixel is closer to the true representation of the anatomic structures because there are fewer tissues in each (thin) volume element. However, thin slices tend to be somewhat "noisier"; the pixels more accurately represent the densities in each of the volume elements,

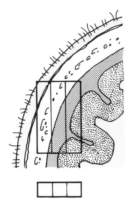

FIG. 3.7. Illustration of "volume averaging." A portion of a *coronal* section through scalp, skull, subarachnoid space, and cortex is shown; the height of three voxels includes several structures and spaces, each with very different densities. When represented in a *horizontal* CT section, the pixels from these voxels show the dominant high density of bone, resulting in a seemingly thick skull.

each of which may be slightly different in density from the adjacent ones. A series of thin slices is of course much more time-consuming than a few thick slices through the same volume; however, a "stack" of thin slices is required for reformatting (see Chapter 7). In some of the thicker, slightly higher sections at approximately this level one may see the *choroid plexus* curve upwards (over the thalamus) within the body of the ventricle, especially after contrast enhancement (Fig. 3.6).

In the *cerebral cortex,* it may be possible to distinguish the *parieto-occipital fissure* (Figs. 3.3 and 3.6). Note that the falx is not present in the middle part of the midsagittal plane in this section (see the midsagittal section, Fig. 3.2, for an explanation of this finding). In contrast-enhanced scans, the branches of the *anterior cerebral arteries* may be seen as small areas of high density; the large veins posteriorly in midplane may be visible, especially the *great cerebral vein* (of Galen).

A normal, axial MR image at the level of the upper thalamus is shown in Figure 3.9. Note (again) the differences between CT and MR: dense bone (skull) is white on CT scans, black on MR

FIG. 3.8. Illustration of the effect of voxel dimension on "volume averaging." A *coronal* cross-section through anterior horns and caudate nuclei is shown: large voxel size (right) results in a seemingly larger ventricle when the pixels are seen in a *horizontal* cut. A reduction in voxel size (left) results in a more accurate depiction of the size and outline of the ventricle.

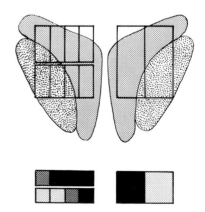

images; the falx and vessels are white on enhanced CT scans, black on (un-enhanced) MR images. Dense bone, air, dura, CSF, and fast-flowing blood in vessels produce little or no signal in Figure 3.9; however, when different parameters are used during the MR procedure, the results are different (see Figs. 3.13A and B).

Human heads vary somewhat in size and shape (Fig. 3.10). The amount of contrast used may vary in the protocol in one radiologic department from that in another. Age is a factor too. It is therefore not surprising that two scans at the same level may look so dissimilar in different persons. Small variations in the section plane may add to the variation between images (see also Figs. 2.10, 2.12, and 2.14).

Altered Anatomy

A clinical example is shown in Figure 3.11; it is a contrast-enhanced scan (the cortical ribbon is clearly seen; the falx and internal and great cerebral veins stand out). The ventricles are

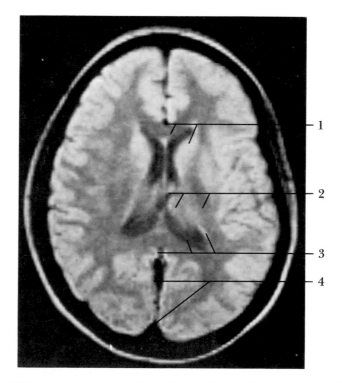

FIG. 3.9. MR image (spin echo) through lateral ventricle and upper thalamus. *1*, Pericallosal artery, genu of corpus callosum, head of caudate nucleus; *2*, internal cerebral vein, upper thalamus, internal capsule; *3*, great vein behind splenium, atrium, tail of caudate nucleus; *4*, straight sinus, superior sagittal sinus.

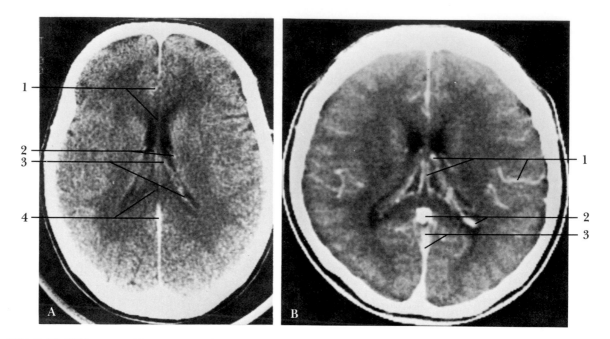

FIG. 3.10. CT images with contrast enhancement. A. 6-year-old. *1,* Irregular pericallosal artery, cavum septi; *2,* internal cerebral veins, thalamostriate vein; *3,* choroid plexus within lateral ventricle; *4,* junction of great vein and straight sinus, splenium. B. 53-year-old, shows the same structures; note the normal difference in ventricular size, shape, calcifications. *1,* Choroid plexus, internal cerebral veins, branch of middle cerebral artery; *2,* calcifications in pineal gland, in choroid plexus; *3,* great vein (of Galen), straight sinus.

too large for this young adult patient, especially the anterior (frontal) horns. There is a prominent linear density in the right hemisphere with one end apparently near the septum lucidum between the two anterior horns. How should these findings be considered? Although the other scans of the series are not given, this image suggests that a shunt was placed in the right lateral ventricle to remedy a pre-existing condition of hydrocephalus (its cause is undeterminable from this single scan). The shunt appears to be functioning, because the gyri are not flattened against the side of the skull, and the sulci are clearly seen in several places.

An abnormal MR image is shown in Figure 3.12: an arteriovascular malformation was seen in an earlier angiographic exam; the study demonstrates that one of the abnormal vessels near the atrium had bled into the right lateral ventricle, spilling over into the left frontal horn.

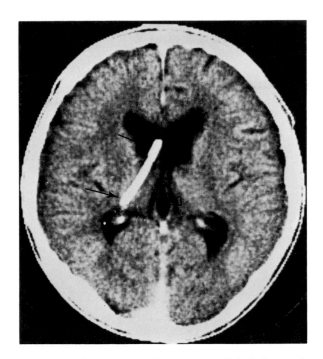

FIG. 3.11. CT image with contrast enhancement, slightly lower than the image in Figure 3.6. Note the configuration of the ventricles, indicating a level through the top of the third ventricle *(arrowhead)* between the internal cerebral veins. All ventricles visible here are considerably enlarged; a shunt *(arrows)* is seen with its tip against the septum.

Effect of Difference in Magnetic Resonance Spin Echoes

Two MR spin echo images at the approximate level of Figure 3.3 are shown in Figure 3.13. In Figure 3.13A the echo delay was 28 msec; in Figure 3.13B, 56 msec. The difference in the images is striking, with better visualization of normal structures in Figure 3.13A. The patient had suffered from chronic hypoperfusion of the cerebrum, hence the so-called "watershed" infarcts near the frontal horns (high signal). An external-to-internal-carotid bypass had been done; the bone flap and soft-tissue swelling are postoperative changes.

The signal in Figure 3.13B is strong for pathologic changes, while the signals for blood vessels are intermediate to low. The two images demonstrate how different MR parameters can produce dissimilar images of the same level in the patient.

Another example of selecting the appropriate settings for better visualization of pathologic changes (this time in a CT scan) is shown in Figure 3.14. The patient, a 32-year-old man, was hospitalized with a history of high fever for about a week, weight loss, and confusion; it was suspected that he had been suffering from septicemia because of an untreated purulent infection of a toe.

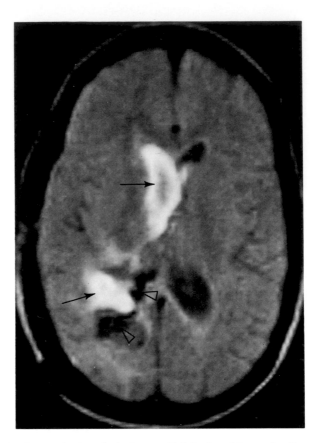

FIG. 3.12. MR image (spin echo). Areas of high-signal intensity (hemorrhage) in right lateral ventricle and right hemisphere *(arrows)*. There is an abnormal vessel pattern with fast-flowing blood in posterior right hemisphere *(arrowheads)*.

The first image, Figure 3.14A, is nonspecific; the contrast-enhanced image, Figure 3.14B, is rather typical of the pathologic condition in the brain, which is a brain abscess.

A 64-year-old patient had suffered a stroke a few months earlier; the CT scan shows infarcts in the distribution areas of the anterior and middle cerebral arteries (Fig. 3.15).

Clinical Cases

CASE 3

A 38-year-old woman gave a 6-month's history of dizzy spells with disorientation; these spells had become more frequent in recent months. She had complained that she often had severe headaches; just a few days ago she had had a grand mal seizure.

NEX: Impairment of memory; slight L papilledema, facial asymmetry; general weakness, symmetrical DTRs. LP: OP, 190. Skull films showed CA^{++} in L hemisphere.

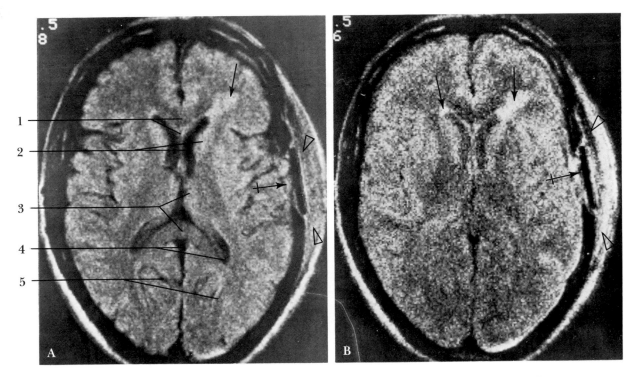

FIG. 3.13. MR images at the level of upper thalamus. A. First echo. *1*, Genu of corpus callosum, septum; *2*, head of caudate nucleus, anterior (frontal) horn; *3*, upper thalamus, splenium with veins averaged-in; *4*, great vein (of Galen), choroid plexus in atrium; *5*, parieto-occipital fissure with vessel, optic radiation. There is a high-signal abnormality *(arrow)* that represents an infarct. There is also an extracranial swelling *(arrowheads)* over a bone flap *(crossed arrow)*. B. Second echo. The CSF has "filled in" with a high signal because of its long T2, the vessels and infarcts are clearly visible, and the background appears "granular" (low signal to noise ratio).

CT Scan (Fig. 3.16): What are your findings? Were the neuroradiologic procedures essential for the DX? Or for the localization of the lesion? What is your DDX?

Three days after brain biopsy, the patient became comatose and died. At autopsy, small hemorrhages were found in the upper brainstem, and the forebrain showed many pathologic features. What was the course of neuropathologic events in the last weeks of life? What is the DX? Where was the primary lesion?

(Discussion of Case 3 on p. 197)

CASE 4   A 66-year-old male alcoholic was found by his landlady on the landing of the stairs. He was stuporous and was aroused only with difficulty. He had bitten his lip and had been incontinent of urine.

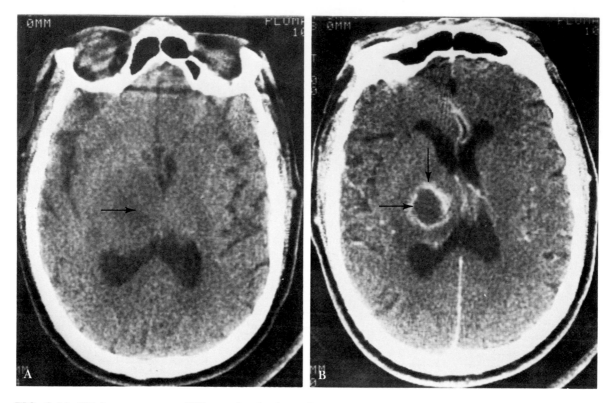

FIG. 3.14. CT images at two different levels through the thalamus. A. Unenhanced image. There is a low-density mass in the right thalamus *(arrow)* causing a right to left shift. B. Higher and contrast-enhanced image. The round low-density area seen earlier now has a ring-like enhancement *(arrows)*.

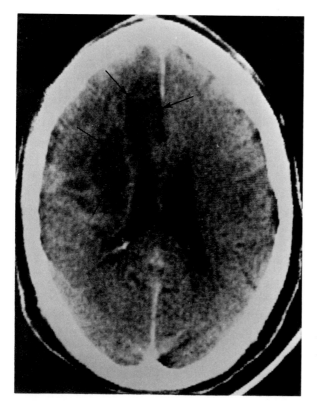

FIG. 3.15. Contrast-enhanced CT image through the lateral ventricle. Several large areas of low density *(arrows)* are seen in the right hemisphere; the right lateral ventricle is slightly compressed. There are linear streak-artifacts in the posterior region.

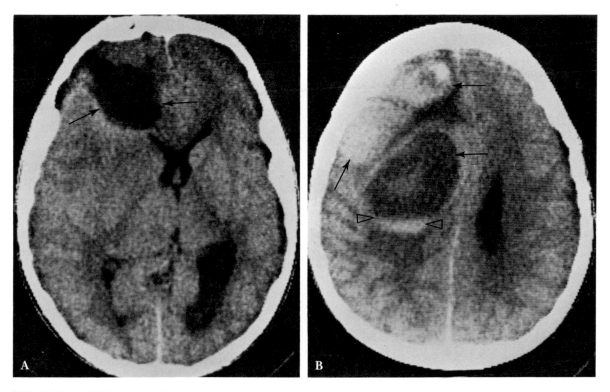

FIG. 3.16. A. CT image without contrast enhancement. A large low-density area is seen in the right frontal lobe *(arrows)*; there is mass effect. B. CT image with contrast enhancement. At the higher level the frontal lobe contains a number of irregular high- and low-density areas *(arrows)*; there appears to be a fluid-fluid level in one of the low-density areas *(arrowheads)*, indicating the cystic nature of the lesion. There is right to left mass effect.

NEX: Several bruises over the lower extremities; swelling on his head. Disorientation, X2. He could talk, when urged, but fell asleep when left alone. Walking was all but impossible. DTRs, NL. L-sided equivocal Babinski's sign. Optic fundi wnl. LP: OP, 180; small number of RBC in all tubes. Patient became increasingly obtunded, and a CT scan was done (Fig. 3.17). What is your DDX? What was the course of neuropathologic events in recent months and in the last few days? What is your DX? What is the anatomic site of lesion?

(Discussion of Case 4 and additional illustrations on pp. 197–198)

Questions   3a. Why can the choroid plexus not be shown in the anterior horn?

3b. Which functional systems pass through the splenium?

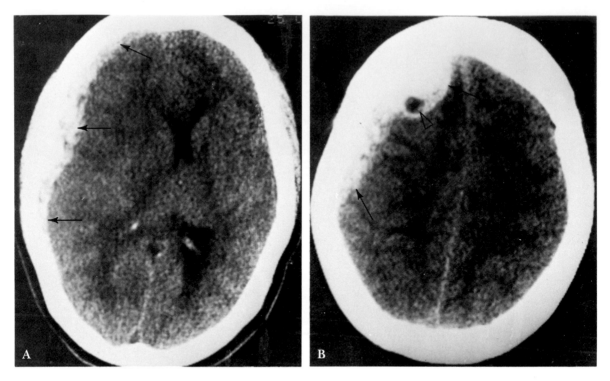

FIG. 3.17. Axial CT images without contrast enhancement. A. A right to left shift is seen, caused by the high-density zone over the right hemisphere, mainly in the frontal region *(arrows);* there is a thickening of the left scalp area. B. A high plane, in which the same high-density zone is noted *(arrows);* there is a round low-density area *(arrowhead).*

3c. Which parts of the corpus callosum should be routinely identified on CT scans?

3d. Parts of which hemispheric lobes can be seen on section B (Fig. 3.1)?

3e. Why is the falx seen discontinued in midplane at the level of Figure 3.3?

3f. Does the choroid plexus have a blood-brain barrier? How can this be demonstrated?

3g. Which fiber systems make up the large area of subcortical white matter mass in Figure 2.8, called the centrum semiovale? (Two of the systems are seen in Fig. 3.3).

3h. Can the superior sagittal sinus be identified in Figure 3.3? Where?

3i. The great cerebral vein (of Galen) is seen to drain into the straight sinus on slice B (Fig. 3.1). What is the other, visible tributary to that sinus?

4. Mid-thalamus *(Anatomic Slice C)*

Normal Anatomy

Anatomic slice C contains a number of additional and important structures and spaces: the *third ventricle* is seen for the first time; the *internal capsule* fibers (continuous with the corona radiata components) course between the *caudate* and *lentiform nuclei* anteriorly as well as the *thalamus* posteriorly. The *insula* and *lateral (Sylvian) fissure* have appeared; the apex of the *tentorium cerebelli* is shown behind the *pineal gland* (Figs. 4.1 and 4.2). The

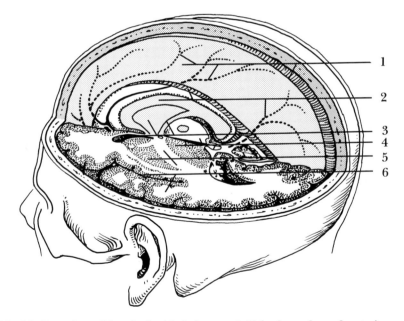

FIG. 4.1. Drawing of level of mid-thalamus. *1*, Falx, branches of anterior cerebral artery, superior sagittal sinus; *2*, corpus callosum, inferior sagittal sinus, branches of posterior cerebral artery; *3*, anterior horn, septum, anterior fornix; *4*, thalamus, third ventricle, pineal gland; *5*, lentiform nucleus, internal capsule (posterior limb), cerebellum (vermis); *6*, lateral (Sylvian) fissure with branches of middle cerebral artery, temporal lobe.

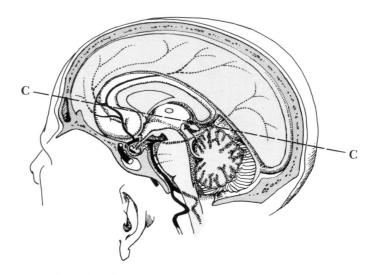

FIG. 4.2. Drawing of midsagittal structures indicating the level of Figures 4.1 and 4.3.

anterior (frontal) *horn* of the lateral ventricle has deepened, and the *atrium* (trigone) is now shown clearly, sometimes (in adult patients) with calcification in the *choroid plexus.*

The anatomic configuration of the structures and spaces at the midthalamic level (Fig. 4.3) is a clinically important one: the small *lenticulostriate arteries* (perforating branches of the anterior and middle cerebral vessels) supply the central area between the frontal horns and the thalamus. Hypertensive bleeding in this area can be explained by the bursting of microaneurysms, especially in the lateral lenticulostriate arteries that supply the putamen, sometimes spreading into the internal capsule, ventricle, or lateral fissure with devastating results. The thalamus is partly supplied by small *thalamic perforator arteries* (off the basilar artery) and partly by the anterior choroidal artery.

The relationships between the three gray masses (thalamus, head of caudate nucleus, lentiform nucleus) and the V-shape of the internal capsule should, therefore, be noted carefully, as this is a clinically important region. Their configuration begins to appear in a previous higher level (Fig. 3.3). The anterior limb of the internal capsule is thinner and carries extrapyramidal and corticopontine fibers. The posterior limb together with the genu is of mixed composition, and essentially continues in lower sections as the cerebral peduncle. The ascending sensory fibers in the medial lemniscus terminate in the thalamus, from where the thalamo-cortical fibers run in the posterior limb; the cortico-bulbar and cortico-spinal fibers run in the genu as well as in this limb.

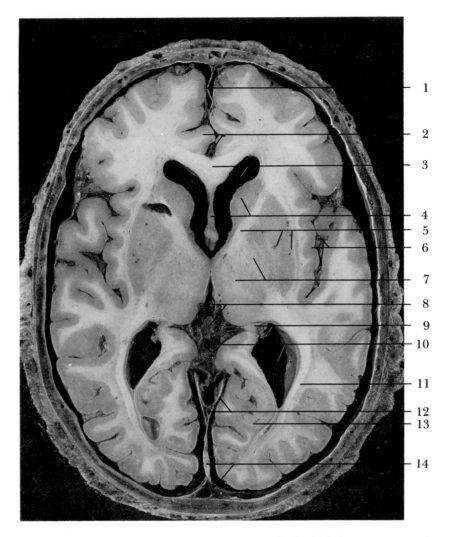

FIG. 4.3. Horizontal anatomic section at the level of midthalamus. *1,* Anterior falx; *2,* cingulate gyrus, branches of anterior cerebral artery; *3,* genu of corpus callosum, anterior (frontal) horn; *4,* septum with anterior fornix, head of caudate nucleus; *5,* anterior limb of internal capsule, lenticulostriate arteries in lentiform nucleus; *6,* insula, branches of middle cerebral artery in lateral fissure; *7,* thalamus, posterior limb of internal capsule; *8,* third ventricle, pineal gland within quadrigeminal cistern; *9,* (posterior) fornix, choroid plexus; *10,* great cerebral vein (of Galen), atrium; *11,* optic radiation; *12,* straight sinus, tentorium; *13,* deep calcarine (visual) cortex; *14,* posterior falx, superior sagittal sinus. (Unsöld, R., Ostertag, C. B., De Groot, J., and Newton, T. J.: Computer Reformations of the Brain and Skull Base. Berlin, Heidelberg, New York, Springer-Verlag, 1982.)

At this time the ventricular pattern (Figs. 2.3 and 4.4) may be reviewed, as well as the position of the third ventricle on the midsagittal section (Fig. 2.5); note the small cistern between third ventricle and the fornix/corpus callosum complex. This CSF-space is the cistern of the velum interpositum, and contains choroidal arteries, the internal cerebral veins, arachnoid, above the habenulae; the cistern opens into the quadrigeminal cistern (see Fig. 7.7).

The fiber systems ascending to and descending from the cerebral cortex converge into the corona radiata and internal capsule, from where connections to the basal ganglia are given off, and other systems added. The main corticospinal or corticobulbar and corticopontine fibers condense below the midthalamic level into the cerebral peduncle (basis pedunculi; Figs. 4.5 and 4.6). The corticospinal system continues through the pons into medullary pyramid, then courses into the spinal cord. Considerable fiber connections exist between the gray masses around the internal capsule, although the masses appear as isolated structures (Figs. 4.5 and 4.6). Note how the lateral ventricles curve around the central gray masses, with the third ventricle lying in midline; lateral to the putamen and the external capsule is found the lateral fissure.

The CT images (Figs. 4.7 and 4.8) should now be studied and compared to the anatomic slice (Fig. 4.3). The low density parallel and far lateral to the *putamen* of the lentiform nucleus is the CSF space of the *lateral (Sylvian) cistern,* in which (after contrast) the branches of the *middle cerebral artery* may be seen. The gray (cortical) region between the cistern and the putamen is the *insula.* At this midthalamic, horizontal level the cortex contains portions of the frontal, temporal, and parietal lobes; in a slightly lower level, the cortex also contains part of the occipital lobe. The midline low-density region contains the *third ventricle* and the cistern of the velum interpositum (in thick slices). These two CSF

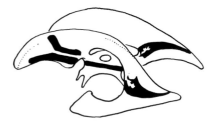

FIG. 4.4. Level of section indicated on ventricular system outline.

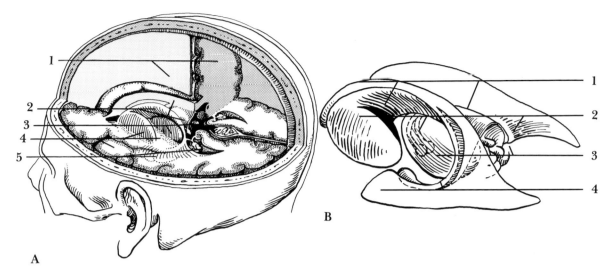

FIG. 4.5. Illustration of the relationships of the central gray masses to the midthalamic axial plane. A. *1*, Coronal plane, falx; *2*, fornix, corpus callosum, caudate nucleus; *3*, quadrigeminal cistern, thalamus; *4*, internal capsule (posterior limb), lentiform nucleus, temporal lobe; *5*, atrium, inferior horn, and hippocampus (below horizontal plane). B. Isolated detail of Figure 4.5A. *1*, Left anterior horn, caudate nucleus, right fornix; *2*, left lentiform nucleus (putamen), right anterior fornix, right atrium; *3*, left thalamus, pineal gland, quadrigeminal cistern; *4*, left inferior horn, tail of caudate nucleus.

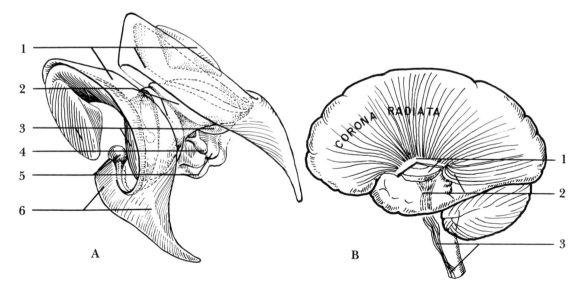

FIG. 4.6. A. Illustration of the relationships of the gray masses to the lateral ventricle (oblique view). *1*, Right lentiform nucleus, right and left lateral ventricles (bodies); *2*, fornices, caudate nucleus; *3*, right thalamus, left thalamus, lentiform nucleus; *4*, pineal gland, hippocampus; *5*, quadrigeminal bodies, termination of tail of caudate nucleus on amygdaloid nucleus; *6*, atrium, left inferior horn. B. Illustration of descending fiber systems in the left hemisphere and brain stem. *1*, Genu of left internal capsule, putamen; *2*, descending fibers in cerebral peduncle, retrolenticular fibers; *3*, left pyramid, lateral corticospinal tract.

spaces are indistinguishable without contrast; after contrast, the *internal cerebral veins* within the cistern may appear clearly (Figs. 4.7 and 4.8; also Fig. 3.6).

In the interhemispheric fissure just anterior to the genu of the corpus callosum the branches of the anterior cerebral artery may be seen. The splenium is no longer visible; behind the third ventricle lies the often calcified pineal gland. The internal cerebral and other veins join the great cerebral vein (of Galen) between the splenium and pineal gland. The CSF-space here has several names (superior cistern, cistern of the vein of Galen): for the sake of simplicity the term "quadrigeminal cistern" will be used (see Figs. 7.7 and 4.2).

A small Y-shaped structure is now visible (after contrast enhancement at the front end of the posterior falx: the short sides represent sections through the upper part of each half of the tentorium (cerebelli), containing between them the very apex of the

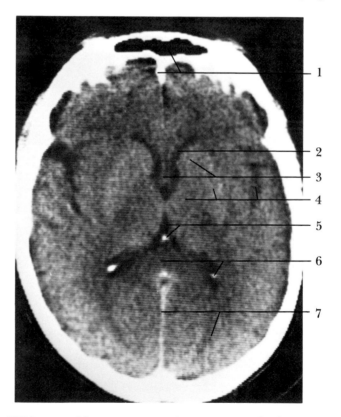

FIG. 4.7. CT image without contrast enhancement at the level of Figure 4.3. *1*, Crista galli, frontal air sinus; *2*, anterior (frontal) horn; *3*, septum (double) with anterior fornices, head of caudate nucleus; *4*, thalamus, lentiform nucleus, lateral (Sylvian) fissure; *5*, third ventricle, pineal gland (with calcium); *6*, splenium of corpus callosum, calcified choroid plexus within atrium; *7*, posterior falx, optic radiation.

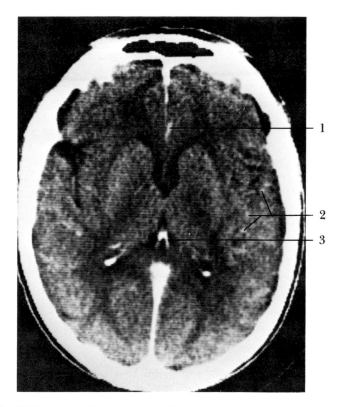

FIG. 4.8. CT image with contrast enhancement at the level of Figure 4.3. *1,* Anterior cerebral artery branch; *2,* branches of middle cerebral artery; *3,* internal cerebral vein.

infratentorial compartment, often called the posterior fossa. The long stem of the Y is the posterior falx (cerebri). In the "seam" between falx and tentorium courses the straight sinus, formed by the confluence of the inferior sagittal sinus and the great vein (of Galen). At this time review the falx and tent as a whole (Fig. 2.2).

An image obtained by the MR method is shown in Figure 4.9. Note again that bone may have two different density signals: white (high-density signal) for compact bone, black (no signal) or gray (intermediate signal) for cancellous or diploic bone. Also visible in this slice are the normal *gray masses* (thalamus, putamen, and caudate nucleus) with the myelinated *internal capsule* (low signal) between them, the genu and splenium anteriorly and posteriorly. The main vessels are quite well seen in this 7-mm-thick section: the middle cerebral artery branches laterally; the veins and sinuses, medially. The pericallosal arteries lie just in front of the genu of the corpus callosum.

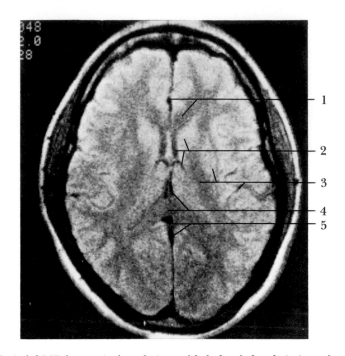

FIG. 4.9. Axial MR image (spin echo) at mid-thalamic level. *1,* Anterior cerebral artery, corpus callosum; *2,* anterior (frontal) horn, thalamostriate vein, caudate nucleus (head); *3,* internal capsule, putamen, branch of middle cerebral artery; *4,* splenium, internal cerebral vein; *5,* great cerebral vein, straight sinus.

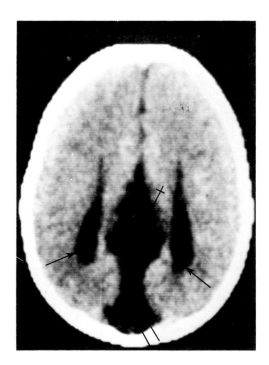

FIG. 4.10. Axial CT image in a 2-year-old child. Lateral ventricles *(arrows);* third ventricle *(crossed arrow);* porencephalic region *(double arrow).*

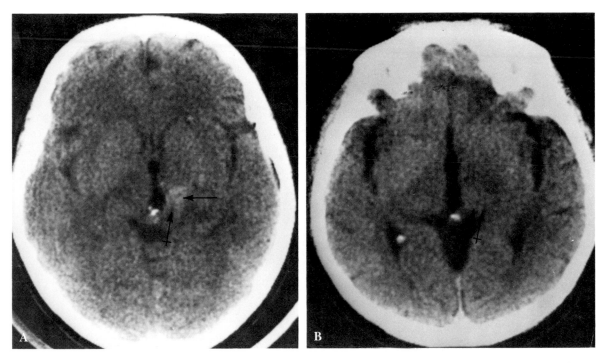

FIG. 4.11. CT images without contrast enhancement at two adjacent levels. A. An area of slightly higher density is seen *(arrow)*, as well as a linear area of low density in the posterior thalamus *(crossed arrow)*. B. A similar low density is seen *(crossed arrows)*.

Altered Anatomy

Several examples of anatomic variants or pathologic images illustrate the clinical importance of this level. In the first CT image (Fig. 4.10, without contrast), the configuration of the ventricular system is quite different from the normal one as shown in Figures 4.3 and 4.4. Note the large third ventricle in the midline and the total absence of the genu of the corpus callosum. The skull is thinner than seen so far because the patient is a 1-year-old child (compare with Fig. 4.7). This image is seen when the corpus callosum is congenitally absent, which results in a large third ventricle that extends higher than normal; the bodies of lateral ventricles do not approach the midplane. This typical pattern of altered ventricular configuration can be readily recognized. The patient has an additional malformation, porencephaly; in such a condition the ventricles communicate directly with the subarachnoid space around the brain.

Two abnormalities are visible in Figure 4.11 (seen without contrast enhancement): a linear low-density area and an unusual high-density area in the left thalamic region. Puzzling at first, these abnormal features become clearer after venous contrast injection (Fig. 4.12). The two abnormalities now are part of a larger

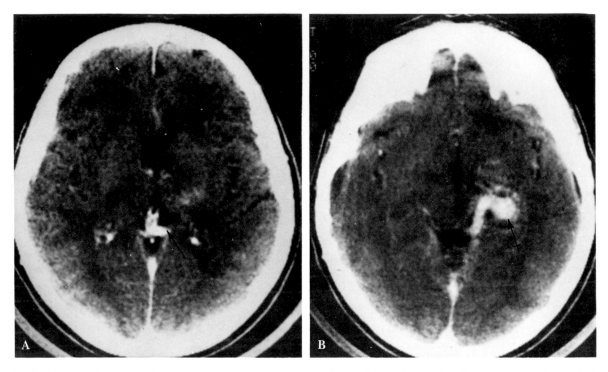

FIG. 4.12. CT images with contrast enhancement at two adjacent levels, 1 day after the images of Figure 4.11 were taken (slight difference in level). A. A large vessel appears near the position of the great cerebral vein of Galen *(arrow)*. B. A somewhat serpiginous high-density area lies in the low-density area seen in Figure 4.11; abnormal vessels are seen in the left thalamus and the region below and anterior to it. Note the round vein *(crossed arrow)*.

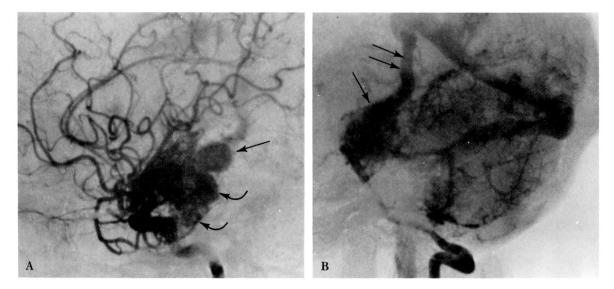

FIG. 4.13. Subtracted angiograms of the patient in Figures 4.11 and 4.12. A. The left internal carotid artery injected with contrast. Note the abnormal vessels *(curved arrows)* and a round, extended early draining vein *(straight arrow)*. B. The left vertebral artery injected with contrast. Note the same round, extended vein *(arrow)* draining into the basal vein *(double arrow)*, then into the great vein, the straight sinus, the confluence, and the transverse sinus, all during the late arterial phase of the angiogram.

entity, a strongly enhancing area with linear and serpiginous densities. How to put all these features together? An angiographic study (Fig. 4.13) shows a thalamic *arteriovenous malformation* to be present with a typical, early-draining vein. The high-density area in Figure 4.11A represents calcification, a not uncommon feature of arteriovenous malformations.

Positioning   The anterior (frontal) horns in Figure 4.14 are asymmetrical in appearance, which may be due to one of several causes: congenital differences between the left and right horns such as in hemiatrophy of the brain (unlikely in this case since the brain and skull are otherwise normal in size); congenital coarctation of part of the anterior horn, so that it has not developed fully; or asymmetrical positioning of the head in the scanner, so that one side is lower and closer to the thinner bottom end of the anterior horn (this cause is unlikely since the image overall seems quite symmetrical, excepting the anterior horns). Small differences between the ventricles and their subdivisions are often noticeable and usually benign in significance. In this case, a small infarct

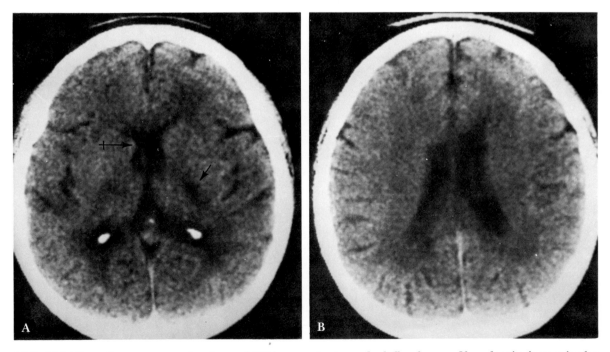

FIG. 4.14. Two adjacent, contrast enhanced CT images. A. A poorly defined area of low density is seen in the left internal capsule *(arrow)*. On both scans there is a striking asymmetry in the ventricles, with a suggestion of abnormal vascularity in the right caudate nucleus *(crossed arrow)*. B. Scans taken 6 months later. Resolution of the small infarct is shown, but there is no change in the ventricular size.

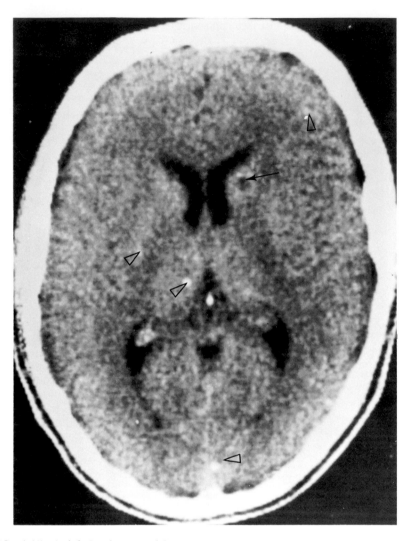

FIG. 4.15. Axial CT image without contrast enhancement. Note the circular low-density area in caudate nucleus *(arrow)* and several small, high-density spots *(arrowheads)* resembling the calcified pineal area.

added to the asymmetry between the left and right anterior horns. Repeat scans showed the asymmetry of the anterior horns to persist, which indicated coarctation as well.

There is one evident abnormality in Figure 4.15, and a few subtle ones. Figure 4.15 is a scan of a white male patient who had been hospitalized with complaints of increasingly severe headaches, periods of fever, and some vaguely defined abnormal body movements. A careful history of the patient indicated that he had visited Mexico and Central America, where cysticercosis is endemic. Blood titers for cysticercosis were measured to be high. The low-density area in the left caudate nucleus was interpreted as an active cyst, while the calcifications were thought to represent dead organisms.

Figures 4.16A and B were taken 1 week apart (both without contrast enhancement). The earlier image shows a poorly defined, low-density area in the right thalamus; there is no mass effect. The later scan better demonstrates the low density, which is round and well-defined. In this case, the diagnosis, an infarct, was confirmed on the strength of a careful examination of the cardiovascular system.

"Look-alikes" It is important to realize that single abnormal scans may look alike, even with a quite different underlying cause (compare Fig. 4.15 with Fig. 4.16B and Fig. 3.14A). Without an adequate history and a careful physical and neurological examination, such "look-alikes" may precipitate errors in radiologic diagnosis. Sometimes a second scan is necessary, with or without contrast, in a different plane, or with special CT methods, such as cisternography, where appropriate (see Chapter 7), or bolus injection of contrast. Other

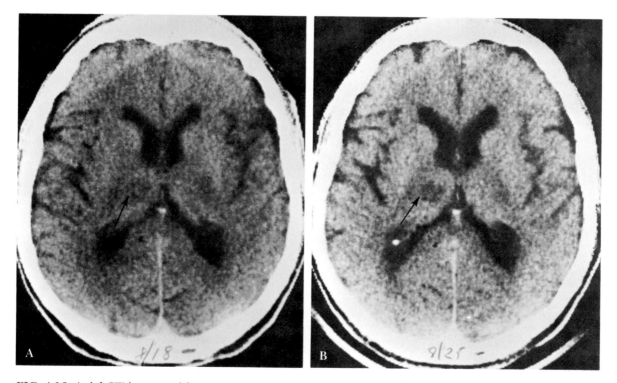

FIG. 4.16. Axial CT images without contrast enhancement, taken a week apart. A. A poorly defined area of low density is seen in the right thalamus *(arrow)*. B. The later image shows the low-density area *(arrow)* more clearly.

methods that may be used are angiography or an MR scan. The pseudodiagnosis of lesions in areas that are close to a rich blood supply, e.g. a "tumor" in a cerebellar flocculus or vermis near the choroid plexus, has been made in the past; both pseudodiagnosis and misdiagnosis should be avoided.

Clinical Cases
CASE 5

A 20-year-old black male motorcyclist was brought to the ER. He had been found unconscious in the street; apparently he had slipped in a curve and hit his head on the curb (no helmet!).

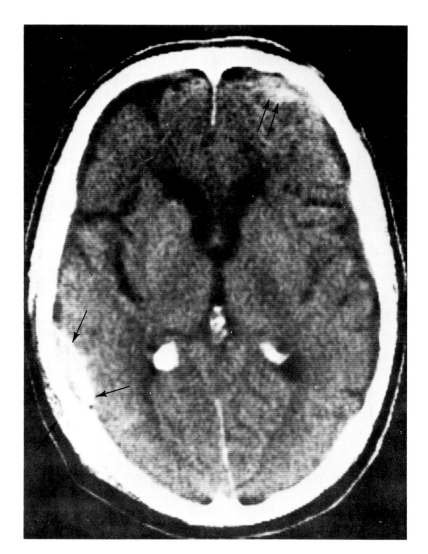

FIG. 4.17. Axial CT image without contrast enhancement at mid-thalamic level. Note the scalp bruise *(crossed arrow)*, the lens-shaped high density *(arrows)* representing freshly clotted blood, and the high density contusion *(double arrow)* on the opposite side ("contrecoup").

While in the ER he became conscious for a while, appeared dazed, complained of HA, then seemed to doze off again.

NEX: No PE, EOMs full, questionable L. VII N. weakness. DTRs lively. BP, 120/90; PR, 75, RR, 14.

What is your DDX at this time? What is your best neuroradiologic procedure now? Would you do an LP? A CT scan was done (Fig. 4.17).

Patient was kept under observation: his BP went up; PR and RR went down. He then underwent emergency neurosurgery. What is the DX?

(Discussion of Case 5 and additional figures on pp. 199–200)

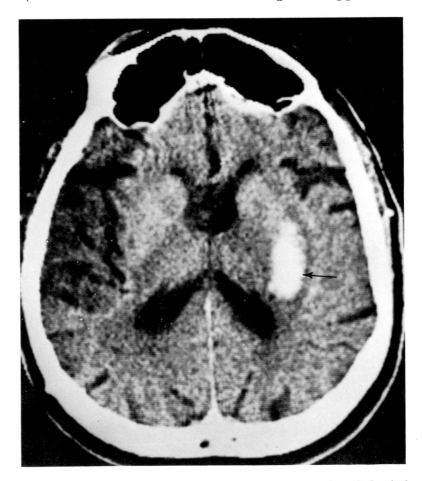

FIG. 4.18. CT image without contrast enhancement at the low-thalamic level (angle of cut is different from the infraorbital base plane). There is a high-density area in the left lentiform nucleus, extending into the posterior limb of the internal capsule *(arrow)*. A large low-density zone in the right temporo-parietal area is seen. The sulci are quite wide (the result of age), and the frontal air sinus is unusually large.

CASE 6   A 59-year-old housewife with known hypertension (230/120) had a sudden episode of L central facial weakness, L hemiplegia, and L loss of sensation; shortly afterwards she lost consciousness. No PE. Tongue deviated to L.

NEX: Flaccid muscles on the L side, no DTRs LUE, increased in the LLE; L extensor plantar reflex.

Where is the lesion? What is your DDX? What neuroradiologic procedure would you prefer to have? A CT scan was made *without contrast* (Fig. 4.18). What is the DX? Which vessels were involved? (Be specific: look at slice C again, Fig. 4.3).

(Discussion of Case 6 and additional figures on pp. 201–202)

Questions   4a. Between which gray (cellular) masses is the posterior limb of the internal capsule situated?

4b. What is the composition of the posterior limb of the internal capsule? Of the anterior limb? Of the genu?

4c. Which three calcified structures may normally be seen on this slice?

4d. The branches of which artery are found in the lateral fissure? In the interhemispheric fissure?

4e. Can the infratentorial compartment (posterior fossa) be seen at all in this (high) section? Why?

4f. Portions of which cerebral lobes may be present in slice C (Fig. 4.3)?

4g. Identify the low density (low signal) crossing the midline in front of the anterior horns (Figs. 4.8 and 4.9).

5. Hypothalamus; Upper Midbrain (*Anatomic Slice D*)

Normal Anatomy

This section lies below the thalamus and cuts across the *hypothalamus* and upper *midbrain;* the plane of section is just above the interpeduncular fossa (Figs. 5.1 and 5.2). The *lateral fissure* is deeper and wider than in previous sections; it will connect with the basal cisterns in the next lower section. In the *fissure* course the main *branches* of *middle cerebral artery.* On the midsagittal plain shown in Figure 5.2, the main stem of the *anterior cerebral artery* is shown, continuing around the genu of the corpus callo-

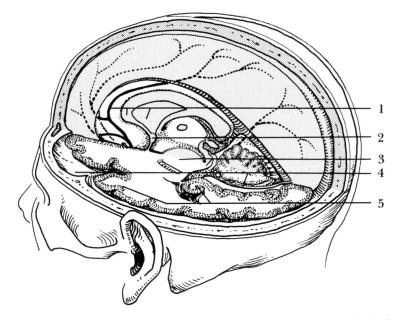

FIG. 5.1. Drawing of the anatomic relationships of level D through the hypothalamus and upper midbrain. *1*, Pericallosal artery, genu of corpus callosum, septum; *2*, anterior commissure, great cerebral vein; *3*, upper midbrain, superior colliculus, cerebellar vermis; *4*, roof of orbit, substantia nigra, tentorium; *5*, temporal lobe, inferior (temporal) horn with choroid plexus, hippocampus.

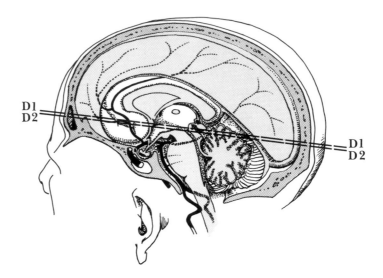

FIG. 5.2. Drawing of midsagittal structures and spaces to illustrate level of slice D.

sum. The frontal air sinus, a variable cavity within the frontal bone is just visible anteriorly in Figure 5.1.

The *frontal lobe* lies just above the *orbital roof* and the *temporal lobe* is continuing into the *occipital lobe.* At the transition area between temporal and occipital lobes, the change from atrium to *inferior* (temporal) horn of the lateral ventricle is cut across. The *substantia nigra,* the *aqueduct,* and the *quadrigeminal bodies* of the midbrain lie in front of the upper cerebellum. Note the *straight sinus* on its way to the confluence with the *superior sagittal sinus.*

Two anatomic images (Figs. 5.3 and 5.4) illustrate the rapid changes that occur in the anatomic relationships in the region of the transition between cerebrum and brain stem. Figure 5.3 is the upper aspect of a slice just above level D; Figure 5.4 is the lower aspect of the same slice, and corresponds to Figure 5.1. Note the changes in the ventricular cross-section (compare Figs. 4.4 and 5.5): the *third ventricle has given way* (in the lower section) to the *aqueduct* and the *lower* and more *anterior* hypothalamic portion of the *third ventricle.* The *atrium* (and occipital horn) in the higher section merges lower and more anteriorly into the temporal (inferior) horn (Fig. 5.4).

The *anterior commissure* lies just above the lamina terminalis, the rostral end of the embryologic neural tube. The *basal ganglia* (caudate, lentiform nuclei) are more compact in Figure 5.4 than in the higher Figure 5.3; similarly, the *lenticulostriate arteries* are not only larger in diameter, but closer together. The *middle cere-*

bral artery branches lie in the lower section, within a less extensive *lateral fissure* (compare Fig. 5.3 to Fig. 5.4). The *thalamic perforators* are a number of *small arteries* seen in the lower thalamic area; these, and the small arteries supplying the upper midbrain, come off the basilar artery in the interpeduncular fossa (see Chapter 6). The shape of the *midbrain* is clearly discernible in Figure 5.4 in its transition with the posterior diencephalon. Figure 5.3 shows how

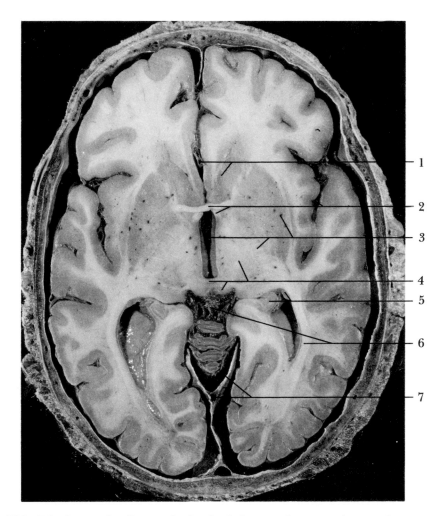

FIG. 5.3. Anatomic slice at the level of the anterior commissure; the upper surface of the slice is shown. *1*, Pericallosal artery in interhemispheric fissure, head of right caudate nucleus; *2*, anterior commissure, anterior fornix, middle cerebral artery branch in right lateral fissure, between insula and temporal lobe; *3*, third ventricle, lower portion of internal capsule, lenticulostriate artery in putamen; *4*, posterior commissure, superior colliculus, lower thalamus plus perforators; *5*, hippocampus, tail of caudate nucleus; *6*, quadrigeminal cistern with vessels and arachnoid trabeculae, right optic radiation; *7*, straight sinus, tentorium.

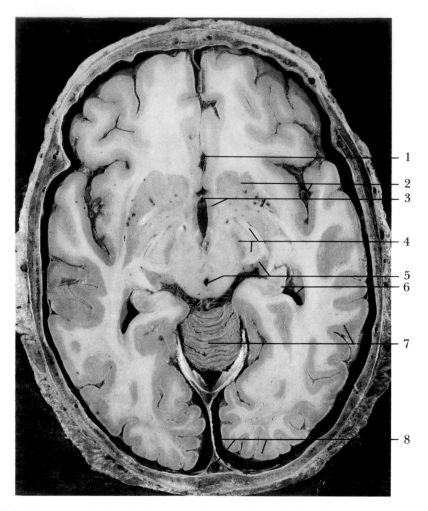

1

2

3

4

5
6

7

8

FIG. 5.4. Anatomic slice D (lower surface) at the level of the lower third ventricle. *1,* Anterior cerebral artery in interhemispheric fissure, middle meningeal artery branch grown within skull; *2,* junction of left caudate and putamen, middle cerebral artery branch within lateral fissure; *3,* lamina terminalis, hypothalamus along lower third ventricle, lenticulostriate arteries; *4,* substantia nigra (upper part), cerebral peduncle, left optic tract; *5,* aqueduct, ambient or perimesencephalic cistern, lateral geniculate body; *6,* hippocampus, beginning of inferior horn; *7,* cerebellar vermis, parietal cortex; *8,* posterior falx, superior sagittal sinus, occipital cortex.

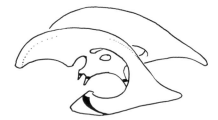

FIG. 5.5. Drawing of ventricular "slice" at the level of Figure 5.4.

the pulvinar of the thalamus lies just higher than the thalamic *geniculate bodies* (Fig. 5.4).

More of the *cerebellum* is seen in the lower section; the shape of the cross-cut *tentorium* is changing from a "V" shape to a more rounded bowl shape. These and other changes in shape at lower levels (see Chapters 6 and 7) are useful landmarks in determining the level of the anatomic section, CT image, or MR image.

Two axial MR images at the transition area between thalamus and midbrain are seen in Figure 5.6. The level of sectioning is somewhat lower anteriorly than in the anatomic slices. The main vessels are clearly seen, especially in Figure 5.6B, where the CSF spaces are not well shown. The transition from posterior limb of internal capsule (Fig. 5.6B, then Fig. 5.6A) to cerebral peduncle (Fig. 5.4) is well demonstrated.

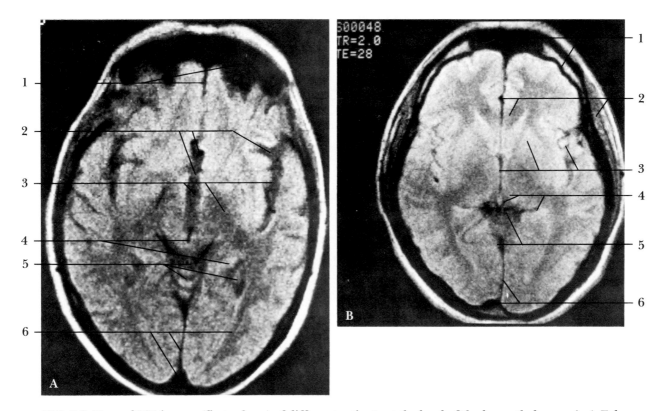

FIG. 5.6. Normal MR images (first echoes) of different patients, at the level of the lower thalamus. **A.** *1*, Falx in interhemispheric fissure, frontal air sinus; *2*, lateral fissure, anterior cerebral artery, lamina terminalis; *3*, branch of middle cerebral artery, cerebral peduncle, third ventricle; *4*, hippocampus, ambient cistern, aqueduct; *5*, choroid plexus in temporal horn, pineal calcification, cerebellar vermis; *6*, optic radiation, superior sagittal sinus, posterior falx. **B.** Slightly higher plane. *1*, Frontal air sinus, skull, (inner table); *2*, anterior cerebral artery branches, corpus callosum, temporalis muscle; *3*, third ventricle, putamen, middle cerebral artery branches; *4*, internal cerebral vein, thalamus, posterior cerebral artery branch; *5*, straight sinus, quadrigeminal cistern; *6*, superior sagittal sinus, posterior falx.

Computed tomography images at this level correspond closely to the anatomic section (Figs. 5.7 and 5.8); in 10-mm-thick sections the interpeduncular fossa may be "averaged in", as well as some stretches of the *major vessels* (Fig. 5.8). Note that a series of CSF-containing spaces is just visible in the midline from front to back: interhemispheric fissure with anterior cerebral artery, third ventricle, aqueduct, quadrigeminal cistern, supracerebellar cistern, and interhemispheric fissure with falx (compare Fig. 5.3).

A midsagittal anatomic section (Fig. 5.9A) demonstrates how the more anterior hypothalamic portion of the third ventricle lies more inferior than the upper end of the aqueduct. A horizontal plane connecting the anterior and posterior commissures (Reid's anthropological base plane) corresponds with an axial plane that is parallel with the infraorbitomeatal base plane; Reid's plane is an approximate separation between the thalamus above and the hypothalamus below. Note the curvature of the aqueduct, a reflection of the embryonic cephalic flexure.

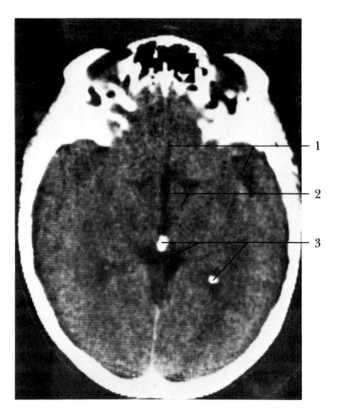

FIG. 5.7. Normal CT image without contrast enhancement, in a plane slightly tilted from that of Figure 5.4. *1*, Interhemispheric fissure space, lateral fissure; *2*, inferior third ventricle, hypothalamus; *3*, pineal calcification, quadrigeminal cistern, choroid plexus calcification in atrium.

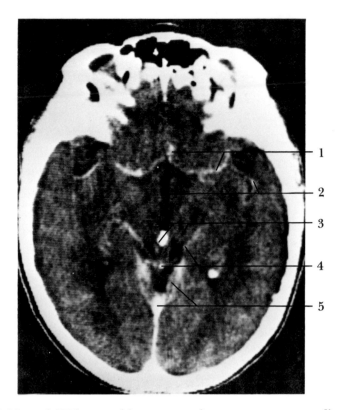

FIG. 5.8. Normal CT image with contrast enhancement, corresponding to Figure 5.7. *1*, Anterior cerebral and communicating arteries, middle cerebral artery; *2*, lower third ventricle, lateral fissure with branch of middle cerebral artery; *3*, beginning of aqueduct, calcium in pineal, upper midbrain; *4*, small vessels in quadrigeminal cistern, posterior cerebral artery; *5*, straight sinus, tentorium.

Venous Drainage of the Brain

An illustration of the venous drainage of the brain is given in Figure 5.9B. The venous channels that lie *on the convexity* of the cerebral hemisphere, the superior sagittal and transverse sinuses (sphenoparietal sinus not shown), join with the deeper venous system at the *confluence*. The *deep veins* (internal cerebral, basal, and other veins) drain by way of the great cerebral vein into the *straight sinus* and confluence. The *cavernous sinus* near the skull base drains into the sigmoid sinus on either end and into the pterygoid plexus (not shown). Most of the venous drainage of the brain is by way of the *internal jugular veins* into the superior vena cava. Note how the ophthalmic veins form a link between the external and internal jugular drainage systems.

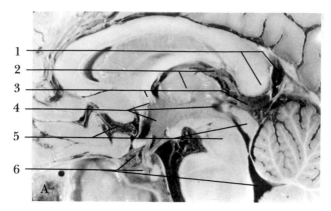

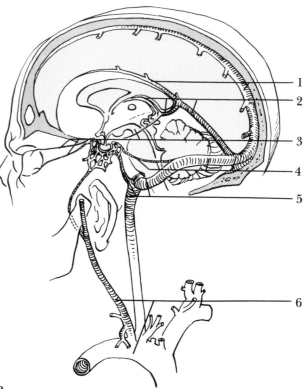

FIG. 5.9. **A.** Anatomic, midsagittal illustration of normal structures in and around the third ventricle. *1*, Great cerebral vein, splenium; *2*, internal cerebral vein, thalamus; *3*, pineal gland, anterior fornix; *4*, posterior commissure, hypothalamus, anterior commissure; *5*, tectum behind aqueduct, midbrain, anterior cerebral artery in interhemispheric fissure; *6*, pituitary gland, suprasellar cistern, fourth ventricle. **B.** View of the venous drainage of the brain. *1*, Inferior, superior sagittal sinus; *2*, internal cerebral veins, great cerebral vein, straight sinus; *3*, ophthalmic veins, cavernous sinus, basal vein; *4*, superior petrosal sinus, transverse sinus, confluence of sinuses; *5*, internal jugular vein, inferior petrosal sinus, sigmoid sinus; *6*, external jugular vein, superior vena cava.

B

Normal Calcifications

Figure 5.10 demonstrates several calcifications that may occur in the brain of an elderly patient (a 66-year-old in this case); these calcifications can be found in the pineal gland, in the choroid plexus, and in the basal ganglia, especially the globus pallidus. While the latter calcification may be present normally, it may also occur in patients with hyperparathyroidism, or after irradiation. There is a low-density area in the right temporal lobe (Fig. 5.10), which is interpreted as an infarct due to the occlusion of middle cerebral artery branches.

Altered Anatomy

A slightly abnormal CT image is shown in Figure 5.11A; note the large irregular area of low density in the left hemisphere. A lower image, Figure 5.11B, shows low-density areas in *both* temporal lobes, with high density (blood? exudate?) in the cisterns surrounding hypothalamus and midbrain. This could have a vascular cause, such as an arteriovenous malformation with infarcts and subarachnoid hemorrhage; however, the bilaterality of the low-density areas tends to argue against it. This patient was sub-acutely dysphasic, drowsy, complained of headaches, ran a temperature, and became quadriparetic all within a month. The diagnosis of this patient was herpes simplex encephalitis, a disease that is accompanied by extensive brain destruction, especially in the temporal lobes.

An even more devastating image is seen in Figure 5.12, a CT scan of a very sick 2-year-old child; a presumptive diagnosis of herpes encephalitis (made on the basis of the CT scan) was confirmed by brain biopsy. The high-density areas, including the midbrain, were then thought to be inflammatory necrosis. This was also seen at autopsy 2 days later.

The CT image shown in Figure 5.13 was puzzling: the 43-year-old patient had been ill with fever, headaches, and muscle weakness for a week before hospitalization. The brain appeared to be swollen, the gray-white matter differences were not seen, and the vessels seemed larger than normal. A presumptive diag-

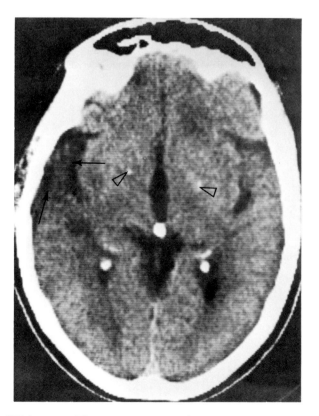

FIG. 5.10. CT image with some contrast enhancement (compare with Figure 5.7). The third ventricle is widened; there are high densities (calcium) in the pineal gland, in the choroid plexus of the atria, and in each globus pallidus *(arrowheads)*. The right temporal lobe contains low-density areas *(arrows)*.

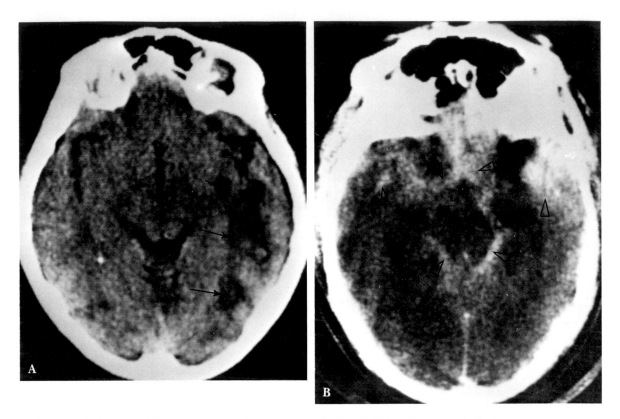

FIG. 5.11. CT images without contrast enhancement at the level of the midbrain. **A.** An irregular area of low density is seen along the left medial temporal lobe *(arrows)*. **B.** One week later, at a lower level, the temporal and frontal low-density areas are now bilateral; there are high-density areas around the midbrain and hypothalamus and in both hemispheres *(arrowheads)*.

nosis of cerebritis was made, and the patient was treated. Angiographic studies were called normal. Three weeks later a repeat scan resembled that of Figures 5.7 and 5.8; the patient had markedly improved, and was discharged a few days later.

Clinical Cases

CASE 7

A 51-year-old white male was admitted with severe headache, nausea, vomiting, and left hemiparesis. Nine mos. PTA Pt noted low back pain. One month later CXR showed coin lesion in left apex. Subsequent thoracic spine film showed decrease in height of T9 vertebra. L upper lobectomy revealed poorly differentiated adenocarcinoma with a positive hilar node. RX: 3000 rads to spine in 14 days and 4000 rads to mediastinum in 4 weeks. Three days PTA Pt developed drooling out of left side of mouth, plus left-sided weakness; 1 day PTA HA, nausea, vomiting; admitted to CRI.

PEX: A thin white man in no acute distress. Skin, NL. No nodes, neck supple. Tenderness at T9 to L1 in back. Decreased breath sounds L upper lobe. Otherwise wnl.

NEX: MS wnl. CNN: L homonymous HAO, papillae flat; full EOMs, no nystagmus; pupils: OS, 2mm; OD, 3mm. Slight L ptosis, normal corneal reflexes. Perhaps L masseter weakness. Other CNs NL. Motor exam showed increase in tone in LUE and LLE and circumduction of gait. Strength, sensation, cerebellar tests reported as normal. L hyperreflexia with L extensor plantar.

Laboratory data: HCT, 39.1; Hgb, 13.0; WBC, 5800, differentiation wnl. ESR, 489. Chest x ray: no new lung lesion, plus degenerative spine lesions. No LP or EEG done.

What neuroradiologic procedures should have been done? What is the rationale for the request? In Figures 5.14A and B the partial

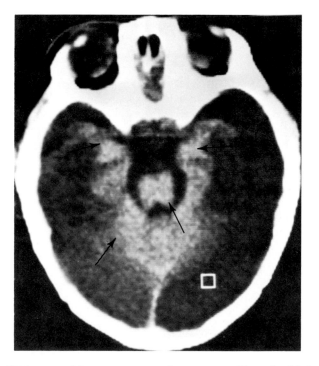

FIG. 5.12. CT image without contrast enhancement. Note the high density in the medial temporal hemispheres and midbrain *(arrows)*; the remainder of the hemispheres, especially the left, shows extensive and irregular low-density areas. The square in the left occipital lobe is a marker for measuring the Hounsfield units of the area enclosed. Note the streak-artifact caused by a dense bony process.

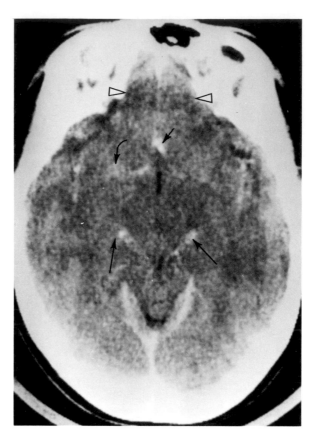

FIG. 5.13. CT image with contrast enhancement at the level of Figure 5.4. All CSF-containing spaces are narrow or not visible. There are several large vessels *(arrows)* and one poorly defined high-density area *(curved arrow)*. Streak-artifacts are present in the left hemisphere, and a "beam-hardening" artifact between the orbits *(arrowheads)*.

results of one imaging procedure are shown. Note the many rounded, high-density areas in the brain (mostly in the territory of which artery?). What is your DX?

(Discussion of Case 7 on p. 203)

CASE 8   A 38-year-old Asian man (right-handed) had been complaining of increasing headache and nausea for several weeks. Pain pills did not seem to have helped him much, but he decided "it would all go away" when he had a good rest. Most recently, he had noted that he seemed unable to look up. His wife then made him see a doctor.

NEX: MS wnl, perhaps slight feelings of depression.

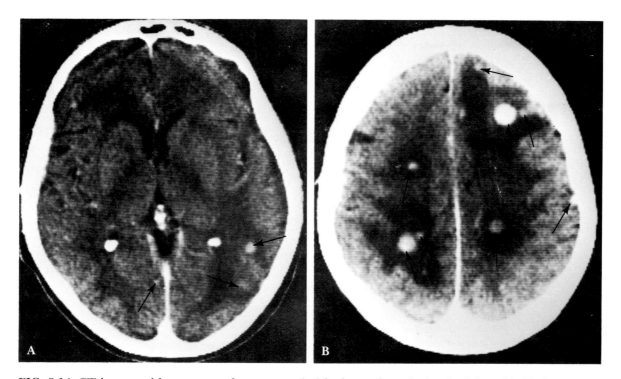

CN:Bilateral PE with some decrease in visual acuity. EOMs restricted in upward gaze. The rest of the examination did not show any abnormalities.

A complete CT scan was done (Fig. 5.15). A contrast-enhancing mass behind the (enlarged) third ventricle was seen. The patient was successfully operated on; 2 months later he had fully recovered.

What was your DDX? Most likely DX?

(Discussion of Case 8 and additional illustrations on pp. 204–205)

Questions
5a. Which major vessels are found anterior to the lamina terminalis (Fig. 5.4)?

5b. Which cerebral lobes are seen, in part, on Figure 5.3?

5c. Which structures and spaces immediately surround the inferior horn seen on Figure 5.4?

FIG. 5.14. CT images with contrast enhancement. **A.** The image is at the level of the mid-third ventricle. Note a few round, enhancing lesions *(arrows)* surrounded by low-density zones. **B.** At least eight such lesions *(arrows)* are seen in the image, a high section; there is some left to right shift anteriorly. The round lesions were not seen on unenhanced scans, but the low-density areas were noted.

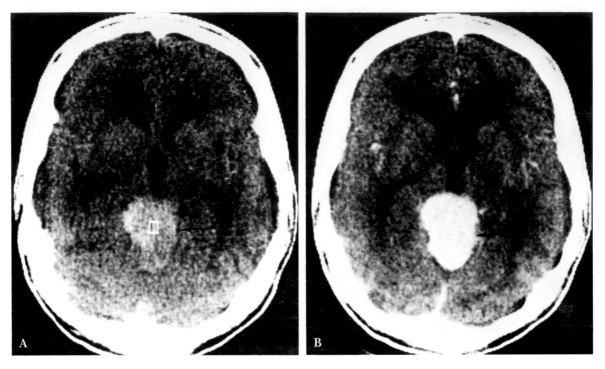

FIG. 5.15. CT images at the level of the third ventricle. **A.** A pear-shaped high-density lesion (*arrow*, with an ROI (Region of Interest) square; Hounsfield unit density, 180) is seen in the nonenhanced scan. The ventricles are enlarged. There are streak-artifacts posteriorly, due to the internal occipital protuberance. **B.** This was taken one day later, after injection of contrast; the mass (*arrow*) is strongly enhancing, and the ventricles appear more dilated.

5d. What lies immediately above the midbrain (Fig. 4.3)? What space lies in front of the midbrain (see Fig. 6.4)?

5e. On what structure lies the occipital lobe?

5f. Which major arteries may be seen on a CT image at the level of slice D (Fig. 5.1)?

5g. Which vessel is the most direct continuation and largest branch of the internal carotid artery? What clinical significance may be attributed to this anatomic finding?

6. Circle of Willis; Suprasellar Cistern (*Anatomic Slice E*)

Normal Anatomy

Anatomic section slice E shows a clear separation between cerebrum and posterior fossa structures (brain stem, cerebellum) (Figs. 6.1 and 6.2). The main landmarks at this level are the *midbrain* with its peduncles and aqueduct; the lower *hypothalamus* (optic chiasma, infundibulum, mamillary bodies); the *subarachnoid space*, called the *suprasellar cistern* anteriorly and the *interpeduncular cistern* posteriorly, with vessels and nerves. Other struc-

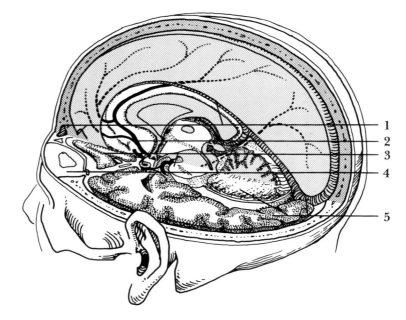

FIG. 6.1. Drawing of level E, through the circle of Willis, suprasellar cistern and midbrain. *1*, Frontal air sinus, crista galli, inferior sagittal sinus; *2*, anterior cerebral artery, optic chiasma, hypothalamus; *3*, gyrus rectus, suprasellar cistern, cerebral peduncle; *4*, upper orbit, uncus, inferior horn; *5*, cerebellum, occipital lobe, confluence of sinuses (previously named "torcular Herophili").

75

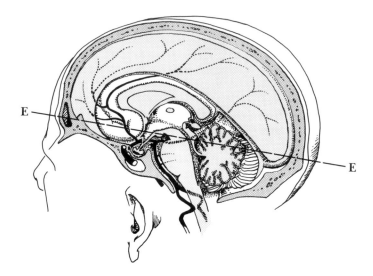

FIG. 6.2. Drawing of midsagittal structures and spaces illustrating level of slice E.

tures and spaces are the most medial portion of the temporal lobe, the *uncus,* lateral to the midbrain, and suprasellar cistern; the *inferior* (temporal) horn of the lateral ventricle curving medially towards the uncus (anterior to it is the amygdala; posterior to it is the beginning of the hippocampus); and the *cerebellum* within the *tentorium.* Note also that this section cuts through the *top* of the *orbit.*

Two anatomic, horizontal sections, a few millimeters apart, illustrate how the main cerebral arteries are related to the spaces around the hypothalamus (Figs. 6.3 and 6.4). In the slightly higher section (Fig. 6.3), the somewhat hexagonal subarachnoid space between *frontal lobes, uncus,* and *midbrain* is called the *suprasellar cistern;* it is filled with arachnoid, *vessels* and contains the lower *hypothalamus.* In Figure 6.4 (slightly lower than Fig. 6.3) this central subarachnoid space has become more pentagonal and contains *chiasma, infundibulum, dorsum sellae, and vessels;* the brain stem cut is across the *upper pons.* Almost the entire *circle of Willis* is visualized when the two sections are considered together. The caliber of the posterior communicating arteries may vary from quite small to several millimeters in diameter. The vessels form a characteristic pattern and therefore are easily identifiable on CT or MR images. Large venous channels, e.g., the straight and superior sagittal sinuses and the confluence, can be readily identified (Figs. 6.3 and 6.4). A cut through the tentorium-falx complex (see Fig. 2.2) at this level looks like a wineglass; in higher sections more like a small cocktail glass (Fig. 5.3), and in low sections it resembles a brandy snifter (Fig. 7.3A).

Arterial Supply to the Brain

The pattern of the main intracranial arteries is shown in Figure 6.5, projected onto the three main fossae of the skull. Note how the *circle of Willis* lies just above the sella turcica of the middle fossa. The *basilar artery* and most of its branches are found in the posterior fossa; above the floor of the anterior fossa course the two *anterior cerebral arteries*.

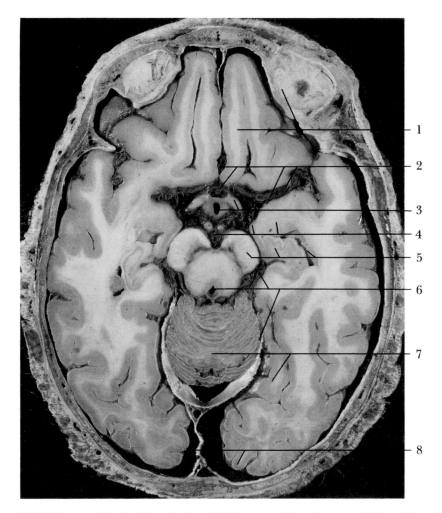

FIG. 6.3. Anatomic slice B at the level of the suprasellar cistern and lower hypothalamus. *1*, Gyrus rectus, upper orbit; *2*, supraoptic recess, anterior cerebral artery, middle cerebral artery in lateral (Sylvian) cistern; *3*, third ventricle (infundibular recess), optic tract, suprasellar cistern; *4*, interpeduncular cistern, uncus, amygdala; *5*, cerebral peduncle, hippocampus, inferior horn; *6*, aqueduct, posterior cerebral artery, tentorium; *7*, cerebellar vermis, medial temporooccipital gyrus; *8*, posterior falx, superior sagittal sinus, occipital lobe.

In Figure 6.6, the main stem vessels are projected on a midsagittal view; the *vertebral arteries* and *carotid arteries* normally are all derived from the aortic arch (only the left internal carotid is shown in its entirety). All main intracranial arteries lie below the brain itself. The *anterior cerebral artery* branches supply the anterior and medial portions of the hemisphere; the *posterior* cerebral artery, after coursing around the midbrain, supplies the occipital and inferior temporal lobes. The *middle cerebral artery* first courses laterally within the lateral fissure, then bifurcates or trifurcates to branch out over the insula, and from there courses over most of the hemispheric convexity (not shown).

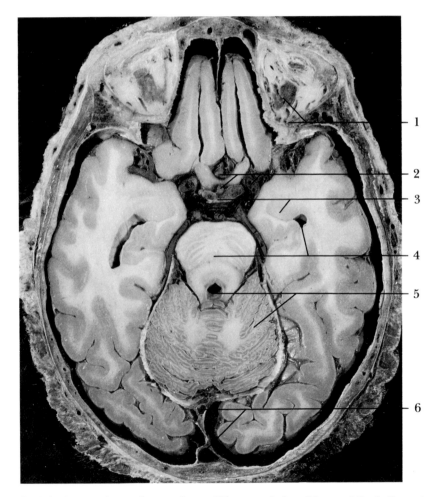

FIG. 6.4. Anatomic section, a few millimeters below Figure 6.3. *1*, Superior rectus muscle, sphenoid ridge; *2*, anterior communicating artery, pituitary stalk behind chiasma, internal carotid artery, *3*, dorsum sellae (slightly displaced anteriorly during sectioning), basilar artery, amygdala; *4*, pons, posterior cerebral artery in ambient cistern, inferior horn; *5*, upper fourth ventricle, cerebellar hemisphere; *6*, straight sinus, superior sagittal sinus.

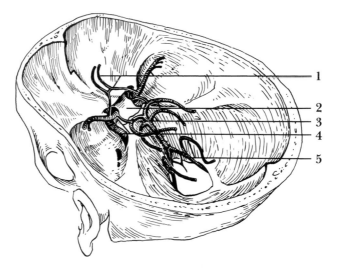

FIG. 6.5. Illustration of the main intracranial arteries projected on a bare skull. *1*, Right anterior cerebral artery (twice), right middle cerebral artery; *2*, sella turcica, right posterior cerebral artery; *3*, basilar artery and right superior cerebellar artery; *4*, internal carotid artery, left posterior communicating artery; *5*, right vertebral artery and right posterior inferior cerebellar artery. Circulus arteriosus (of Willis, not labeled) lies above and around the sella turcica, with the anterior cerebral artery higher than the remainder of the circle.

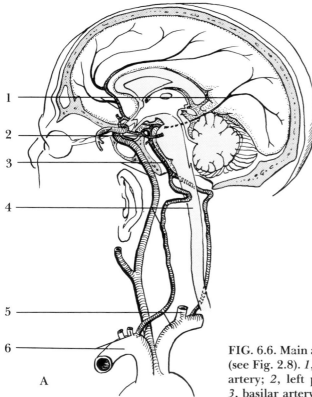

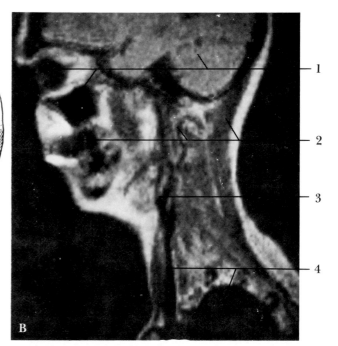

FIG. 6.6. Main arteries supplying the brain. **A.** Illustration, not to scale (see Fig. 2.8). *1*, Right posterior cerebral artery, right anterior cerebral artery; *2*, left posterior cerebral artery, left middle cerebral artery; *3*, basilar artery, left internal carotid artery; *4*, spinal cord, left vertebral artery; *5*, right brachiocephalic artery, right common carotid artery; *6*, left subclavian artery, left common carotid. **B.** Parasagittal MR image (spin echo). *1*, Globe within orbit, maxillary air sinus, cerebellum; *2*, teeth, vertebral artery, trapezius muscle; *3*, carotid bifurcation; *4*, internal jugular vein, lung.

Magnetic Resonance Signals from Vessels

A left parasagittal MR image, which shows some of the stem-vessels, illustrates the anatomic relationships in vivo (Fig. 6.6B). Note how the non-contrast-enhanced, fast blood flow (no signal) makes the vessels stand out from the surrounding tissues. Turbulences within the flowing blood, partial occlusion of the vessel, or atheromatous changes in the vessel wall all may cause a higher-than-normal signal when the appropriate MR echo time is selected (Figs. 6.7A and B).

The normal CT appearance at this level is seen in Figures 6.8 and 6.9. Note how the brain structures, dura folds, and portions of the skull base are separated by cisterns in which the vessels are clearly seen after contrast enhancement. The entire circle of Willis may be seen in thick CT sections, especially if there is slight upward angulation of the plane of section (Fig. 6.10). The posterior communicating artery is often too small to be identified with certainty.

Cisternography

The normal pattern of the cisterns and vessels at the base of the brain is shown in Figures 6.11, 6.12, and 7.7; these CSF-containing, communicating spaces are local, named dilations of the subarachnoid space and therefore display a low density on CT images. At this level the cisterns contain many large, easily identifiable vessels. The cisterns themselves can be readily displayed on CT images by injecting a water-soluble contrast medium into the subarachnoid space, usually by lumbar puncture. If the patient is tilted head down, and this procedure is followed by prone-supine

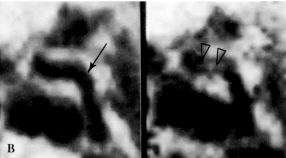

FIG. 6.7. Parasagittal MR (spin echo) images of the carotid siphon. **A.** *1,* Skull, tentorium, lateral ventricle; *2,* cerebellar tonsil, siphon of internal carotid artery, sphenoid air sinus. **B.** An enlargement of the siphon region showing the effect of different echo delay times. No signal in the internal carotid artery, with a 28 ms echo time *(arrow)*; turbulence or atherosclerosis with a 56 ms echo time *(arrowheads).*

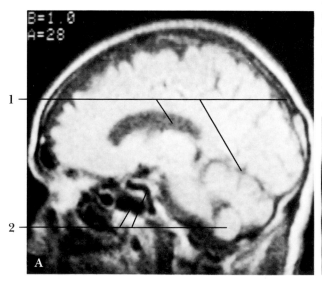

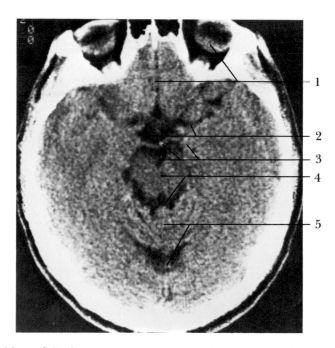

FIG. 6.8. Normal CT image without contrast enhancement. *1*, Interhemispheric fissure, orbit; *2*, suprasellar cistern, infundibulum, lateral (Sylvian) cistern; *3*, interpeduncular cistern, head of basilar artery, uncus; *4*, midbrain, quadrigeminal cistern; *5*, cerebellum, supracerebellar cistern.

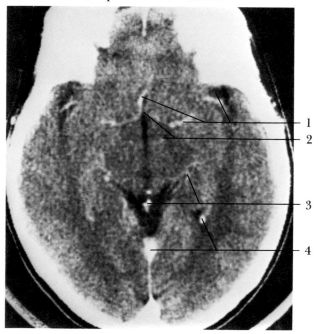

FIG. 6.9. Normal CT image with contrast enhancement, in an axial plane slightly different from that of Figure 6.5. *1*, Anterior cerebral artery, middle cerebral artery (twice); *2*, anterior communicating artery, posterior cerebral artery; *3*, internal cerebral veins, posterior cerebral artery; *4*, straight sinus, choroid plexus with calcium in atrium.

rotation, the contrast mixes more or less evenly with the CSF. Computed tomographic images thus obtained show characteristic, high-density cisternal spaces, and are called *cisternograms* (Fig. 6.12). These images may be used to define normal and pathologic masses more clearly within the cisterns. The procedure causes severe, temporary side effects in some patients; it should not be done without proper indication.

Axial MR images at the level of the circle of Willis are shown in Figures 6.13 and 6.14. The first pair demonstrates the striking differences that occur between two images when the echo delay times are different: in Figure 6.13A (56 ms), the vessels stand out clearly and there is little detail discernible in the brain itself; in Figure 6.13B (28 ms), the vessels within the higher signal CSF spaces are difficult to distinguish, although there is more detail visible in the brain.

There are some differences in orientation of plane of section between Figures 6.14A and B; in both images the vessels of the circle of Willis, part of the posterior cerebral arteries, and the

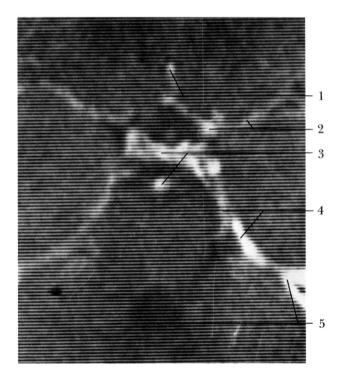

FIG. 6.10. Detail of normal CT image with contrast enhancement, in an axial plane slightly different from that of Figure 6.5. *1*, Anterior communicating artery, anterior cerebral artery; *2*, Internal carotid artery, middle cerebral artery; *3*, dorsum sellae, basilar artery; *4*, posterior cerebral artery, calcified, free edge of tentorium; *5*, fourth ventricle, petrous pyramid of temporal bone.

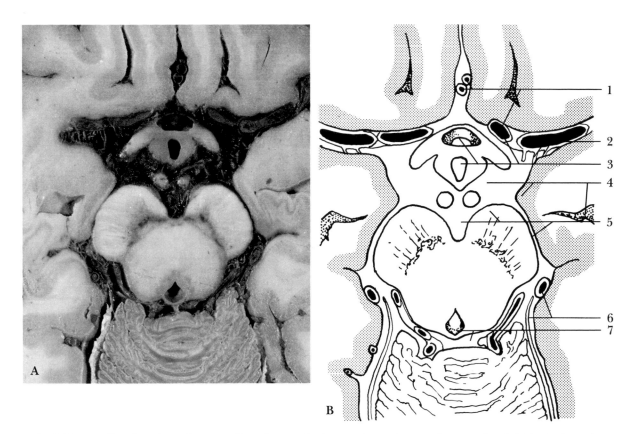

FIG. 6.11. Details of region of suprasellar cistern. **A.** Anatomic section. **B.** Key to Fig. 6.11A. *1*, Anterior cerebral artery (both); *2*, middle cerebral artery, lateral lenticulostriate arteries; *3*, third ventricle recesses, internal carotid artery; *4*, suprasellar cistern, uncus, inferior horn; *5*, interpeduncular cistern, cerebral peduncle, ambient cistern, *6*, tentorium, posterior cerebral artery; *7*, aqueduct, quadrigeminal cistern, superior cerebellar artery. (Fig. 6.11A from Unsöld, R., Ostertag, C. B., De Groot, J., and Newton, T. H.: Computer Reformations of the Brain and Skull Base. Berlin, Heidelberg, New York, Springer-Verlag, 1982.)

sinuses are clearly visible. The pixel size in Figure 6.14A is larger, and the parameters of MR excitation are different than those in Figure 6.14B. The anatomic detail of Figure 6.14A is impressive, and is comparable with that in a CT image (Fig. 6.9), possibly even better.

Altered Anatomy

Two patients with basal meningitis (associated with tuberculosis) are seen in Figure 6.15. The images in these cases look similar to the cisternograms of Figure 6.12; however, the cisterns are filled with high-density infectious matter rather than with an introduced contrast medium. There is evidence of so-called "communicating" hydrocephalus.

Another example of high density in the CSF spaces is seen in Figure 6.16A. In addition, extensive high-density areas are present in the left frontal and temporal lobes. The diagnosis? Subarachnoid hemorrhage and intracerebral hemorrhage from left temporal lobe arteriovenous malformation.

Two months later, the blood had been spontaneously reabsorbed and, the cistern cleared, the underlying arteriovenous malformation is visible (Fig. 6.16B). (This fortuitous turn of events is not always the case.) An MR image that resembles Figure 6.16B is seen in Figure 6.17. However, this patient had suffered from several transient ischemic attacks; the image represents an infarct with surrounding edema.

In Figure 6.18, a partially thrombosed giant aneurysm of the anterior communicating artery is seen together with the main cerebral vessels. Rupture of such an aneurysm, although not common when thrombosed, could produce a picture similar to that of Figure 6.16A.

The difference between an unenhanced CT image and a CT cisternogram with bone-window settings is shown in Figures 6.19A and B; in both images the cisterns are seen clearly, as well as the aqueduct and lower third ventricle. The patient was a 34-year-old man suffering from a drug overdose. Note the atrophy of

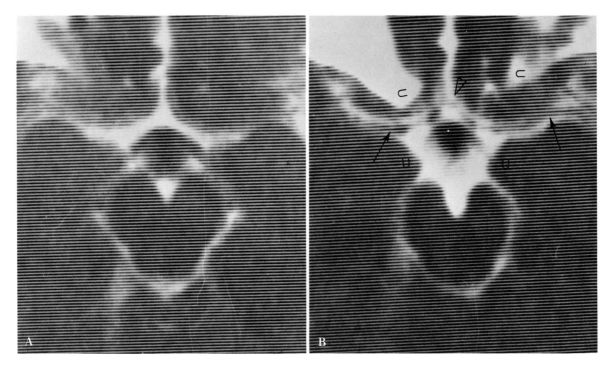

FIG. 6.12. Normal CT cisternograms, at slightly different levels. **A.** The pattern of cisterns is comparable to that in Fig. 6.11.; the vessels are not very clearly seen. Note the low density of the third ventricle (no contrast). **B.** In the slightly lower image, the middle cerebral arteries *(arrows)* and anterior cerebral arteries are seen, as well as the anterior communicating artery *(arrowhead)*; *U* = uncus, *C* = anterior clinoid process.

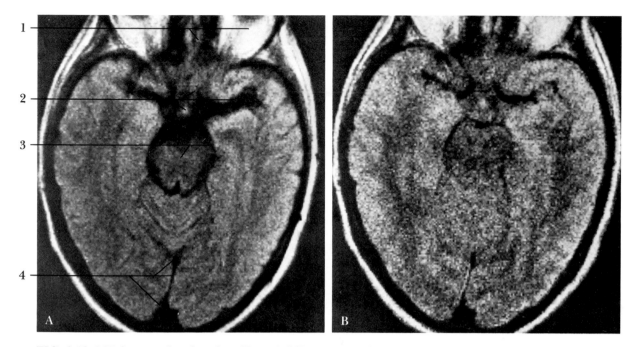

FIG. 6.13. MR images showing the effect of different echo times. **A.** First echo. The CSF has a low-signal intensity that is making the vessels (no signal) poorly visible. *1*, Gyrus rectus, orbit; *2*, infundibulum, anterior cerebral artery, middle cerebral artery; *3*, brain stem, basilar artery, posterior cerebral artery; *4*, posterior falx, straight sinus, superior sagittal sinus. **B.** Second echo. Most of the circle of Willis is clearly outlined; the cisterns have a higher signal than those seen in Figure 6.13A because of the long T2 of CSF. Details of brain less clear.

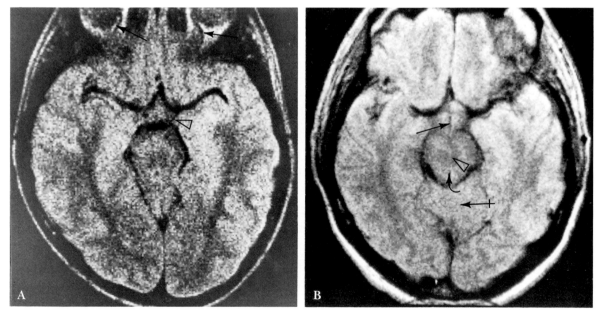

FIG. 6.14. MR images (spin echoes) showing the main arteries in two different patients; the plane of section is not the same. **A.** Second echo. The superior ophthalmic veins are seen *(arrows)* as well as the left posterior communicating artery *(arrowhead)*. **B.** More advanced technique. The vessels, third ventricle *(arrow)*, red nuclei *(arrowhead)*, aqueduct *(curved arrow)*, and cerebellum *(crossed arrow)* are readily identified.

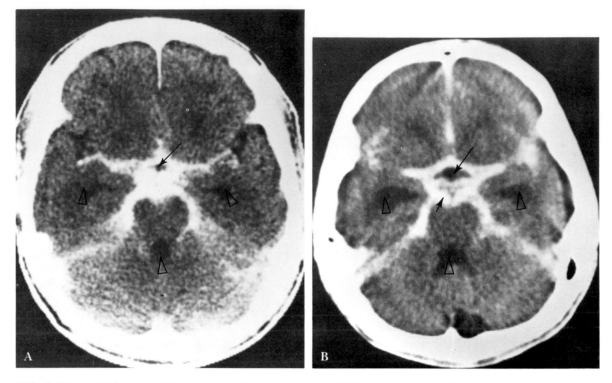

FIG. 6.15. **A.** CT images with contrast enhancement (two different patients). The hypothalamus *(arrow)* is seen surrounded by high densities filling the basal cisterns (compare Fig. 6.12A); the upper fourth ventricle and temporal horns are dilated *(arrowheads)*. **B.** The bifurcation of the basilar artery into two posterior cerebellar arteries is seen as a negative outline *(short arrow)*.

the superior vermis, a finding consistent with the patient's concurrent chronic alcoholism.

Clinical Cases

CASE 9

A 63-year-old white man had been in good health until 6 months previously when a transient, mild R arm and face weakness occurred. This was followed in the next several months by three or four similar TIAs. After the last attack, the weakness persisted; the patient was admitted to a hospital. The diagnosis of arteriosclerotic cerebrovascular disease was made. A CT was scheduled for the next day.

The next morning the patient was found to have had a stroke: complete RUE and RLE paralysis, head deviated to the L. He developed respiratory stress and became comatose. A CT scan was done (Fig. 6.20). What are your findings? What is your DX?

(Discussion of Case 9 and additional illustrations on p. 206.)

CASE 10

A 53-year-old man collapsed at work, complained of a bad HA,

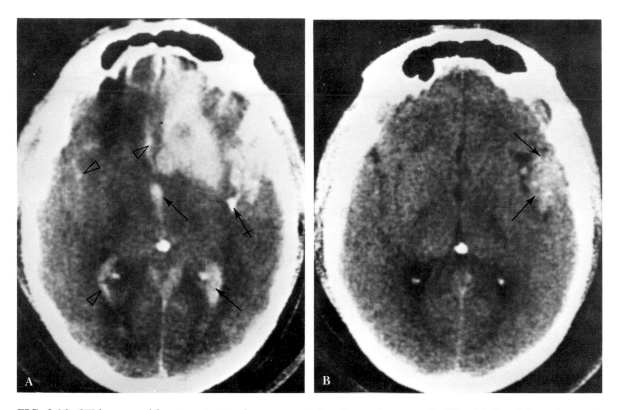

FIG. 6.16. CT images without contrast enhancement taken 2 months apart. **A.** The third and lateral ventricles *(arrows)*, the cisterns of the right lateral fissure and the interhemispheric fissure contain high densities *(arrowheads)*. There is a left to right shift anteriorly. A calcified structure *(crossed arrow)* and an extensive high-density mass are seen in the left fronto-temporal region. All high densities were interpreted as clotted blood. **B.** In the later image, the cisterns have a normal low-density appearance; a partly calcified high-density mass is seen in the left temporal lobe *(arrows)*.

and felt sick. In the ER he was found to be stuporous. PR, 65; BP, 200/110. RR slow. R PE (questionable), L could not be evaluated. Both plantar responses were extensor. There was considerable neck stiffness. A subhyaloid hemorrhage was noted later in the L eye. Also noted was drooping of the R side of the mouth; there was some increase in body temperature.

What is your DX? Would you do an LP? If so, what would you most likely find? What neuroradiologic procedure do you think should be done?

A CT scan was done without contrast enhancement (Fig. 6.21). What are your findings? What is your DX now?

(Discussion of Case 10 on p. 207.)

CASE 11   A 19-year-old black man had complained of mild headaches and decreased vision over a period of several months. He had had

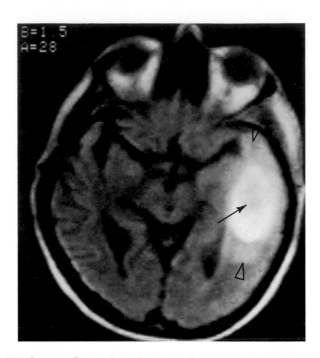

FIG. 6.17. MR image (first echo) showing a large, oval, high-signal area (short T1: blood) in the left temporal lobe *(arrow)*, surrounded by a zone of less intensity *(arrowheads)*, probably edema. There is little mass effect at this level, more in a higher section.

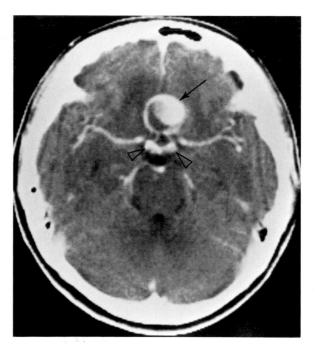

FIG. 6.18. CT image with contrast enhancement at the level of the circle of Willis. A large aneurysm of the anterior communicating artery is seen *(arrow)*, partly thrombosed. Most of the circle is seen; the large dorsum sellae is volume-averaged-in *(arrowheads)*.

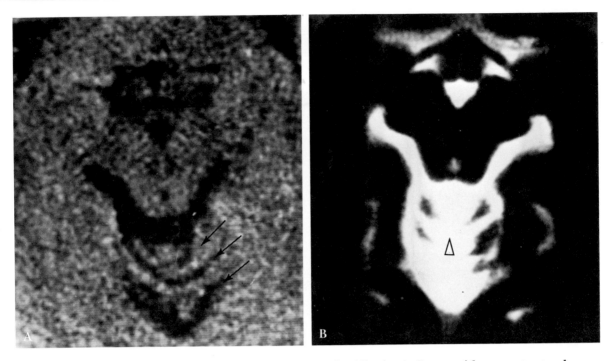

FIG. 6.19. CT images at the level of the hypothalamus and midbrain. **A.** Image without contrast enhancement, showing a normal pattern of cisternal spaces; the folia of the anterior vermis are separated by widened sulci *(arrows).* **B.** A cisternogram was done with clear demonstration of the normal and abnormal CSF spaces; the anterior vermian atrophy is striking *(arrowhead).*

a traffic accident because he had not seen a car coming from the right. Neurologic examination in the hospital revealed a bitemporal HAO, flat optic discs, and slightly increased DTRs. A CT scan was done, first without, then with contrast enhancement (Figs. 6.22A and B). What is your DX?

(Discussion of Case 11 and additional illustration on p. 208.)

Questions

6a. Which CSF spaces can you identify and name in Figures 6.15A and B?

6b. What are the major causes of subarachnoid hemorrhage? How would such a bleeding appear on CT images?

6c. Normally, the tips of the inferior (temporal) horns of the lateral ventricles are not well seen on CT images; what could a clearly identifiable inferior horn, on one side only, signify?

6d. What is the CT density of the optic nerves and chiasma? Is it higher or lower than the CT density of the subarachnoid space?

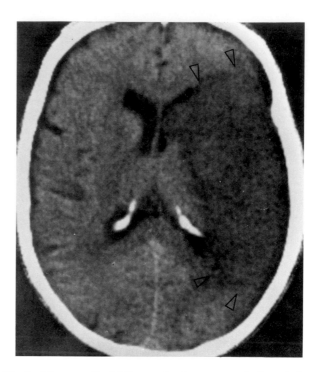

FIG. 6.20. Typical image of middle cerebral artery occlusion. A large low-density area (infarct) is seen in the left hemisphere *(arrowheads)*, consistent with the distribution area of the middle cerebral artery; the anterior cerebral artery and posterior cerebral artery territories are intact.

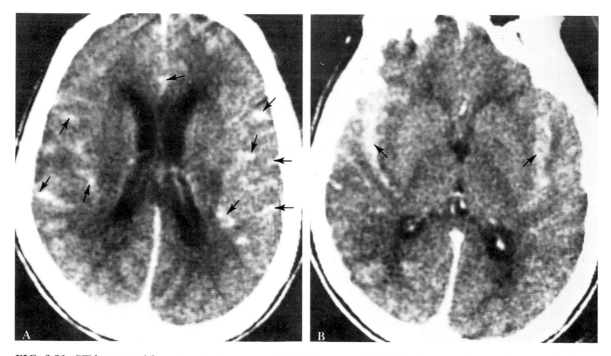

FIG. 6.21. CT images with contrast enhancement. **A.** Numerous high-density areas *(arrows)* are seen in both hemispheres; the lateral ventricles are larger than normal. **B.** These density areas are also seen in the lateral fissures and sulci *(arrows)*.

6e. How could one, theoretically, clearly outline the chiasma, e.g., in cases in which the subarachnoid space was isodense with it, due to aneurysmal "leaking"?

6f. Which cerebral lobes are present at this level of slice E (Fig. 6.3)?

6g. In clinical cases with a probable vascular cause, when would intravenous contrast be used? When would it *not* be used? When would it even be contraindicated (CT examination mode)?

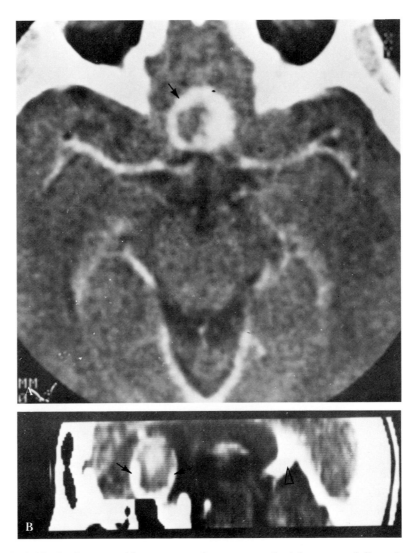

FIG. 6.22. CT images with contrast enhancement. **A.** A large, partially enhancing mass *(arrow)* is seen at the location of the anterior communicating artery. **B.** A midsagittal reformation confirms the location of the mass *(arrows)* in front of the third ventricle; the great cerebral vein *(arrowhead)* and straight sinus are visible.

7. Pituitary Region; Coronal Planes (*Anatomic Slice F*)

Normal Anatomy

Anatomic section slice F is just below the level of the supra-sellar cistern (Figs. 7.1 and 7.2). It cuts through the *orbit, pituitary* region, *pons,* and *fourth ventricle.* The *temporal lobe* and its ventricular horn lie lateral to the dura compartment called *cavernous sinus,* (through, or along, which are four cranial nerves, the internal carotid, and venous channels [see Fig. 7.3]). In the *sella turcica,* the *pituitary* gland lies below the diaphragma sellae (a dura fold of variable extent) and just above the *sphenoid air sinus.* The sella is "hemmed in" between bony processes (*anterior and poste-*

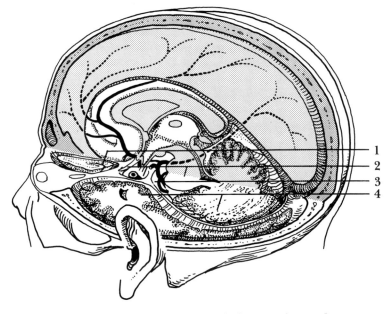

FIG. 7.1. Drawing of level F, through the pituitary region and upper pons. *1,* Gyrus rectus (frontal lobe), anterior communicating artery; *2,* left optic nerve, sella turcica, pons; *3,* (pre) pontine cistern with vessels, upper fourth ventricle, confluence of sinuses; *4,* uncus of temporal lobe, cerebellar hemisphere.

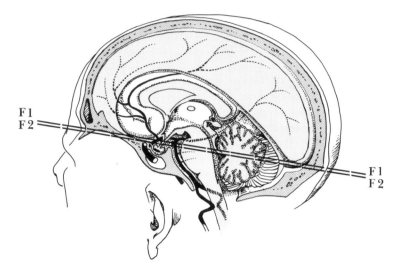

FIG. 7.2. Drawing of midsagittal structures and spaces illustrating level of slice F.

rior clinoids, dorsum, and *tuberculum sellae)* and interconnected dura folds.

Just behind the dorsum sellae (part of the clivus) is found the *pontine cistern* with the *basilar artery* and its branches. Behind the pons the *fourth ventricle,* part of the vermis, and *cerebellum* may be seen, as well as the *confluence sinuum* (sometimes the cut is not exactly through the confluence; however, portions of the main venous sinuses are usually seen).

Anatomic sections just above the sella turcica (Fig. 7.3A) and through the pituitary gland (Fig. 7.3B) illustrate the rapid change in configuration that occurs near the base of the brain. The *vessels* (anterior cerebral artery, posterior cerebral artery, and basilar artery) and *bony landmarks* (dorsum sellae, crista galli, clinoid processes) can be readily identified. The *cerebral structures* and *spaces* (amygdala, hippocampus, temporal horn) lie lateral to the *cavernous sinuses,* while the *pons* and *fourth ventricle* are found behind the sella.

Coronal Sections

An anatomic coronal section through the head shows most of the cerebral hemispheres located above the pituitary/cavernous sinus compartment, and the nasal and oral cavities below (Fig. 7.4). Note how the *temporal lobes* here lie deep to the *lateral fissure* (or Sylvian cistern), lateral to the cavernous sinuses. The suprasellar cistern is traversed by the *internal carotids, infundibular stalk,* and *optic chiasma.*

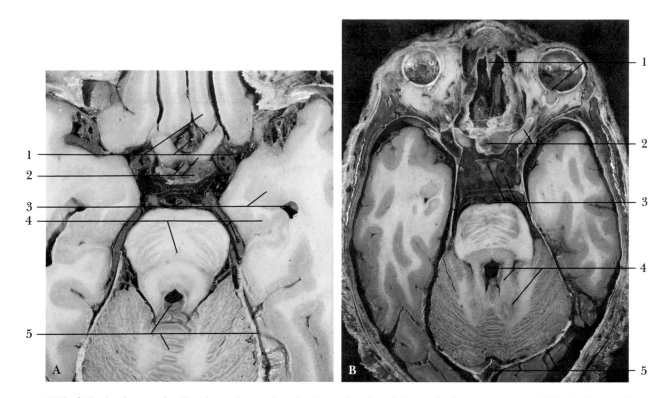

FIG. 7.3. **A.** Anatomic slice just above the pituitary gland and through the upper pons (F1). *1*, Internal carotid artery, anterior communicating artery, gyrus rectus; *2*, dorsum sellae, left optic nerve, pituitary stalk; *3*, temporal horn, amygdala, basilar artery; *4*, hippocampus, left posterior cerebral artery, pons; *5*, tentorium, upper vermis, upper fourth ventricle. **B.** Slightly lower anatomic section at pituitary level (F2). *1*, Crista galli, optic papilla; *2*, tuberculum sellae, anterior clinoid process, left optic nerve; *3*, basilar artery, pituitary, intracavernous internal carotid artery; *4*, fourth ventricle, superior cerebellar peduncle, dentate nucleus; *5*, straight sinus, tentorium.

     The normal axial CT appearance at this level is shown in Figures 7.5A and B. The cisterns around the midbrain are clearly seen in Figure 7.5A, even without cisternography. The cavernous sinuses are seen flanking a partially "empty" sella; the dorsum sellae is not entirely compact. The sphenoid air sinus lies in front of the pituitary fossa, and usually extends below the sella (see Fig. 5.9). There are streak-artifacts visible in the temporal pole region, more strikingly seen in Figure 7.5B, in which the pituitary fossa appears filled with the gland. Possibly the artifacts are more evident because the patient in Figure 7.5B appears to have denser bone, e.g., in the dorsum sellae. The cisterns are less well seen than in Figure 7.5A. Note how the posterior fossa elements within the petrous pyramids are more extensively seen in Figure 7.5B, although the anterior portion of the image (crista galli and olfactory bulbs) lies at about the same level as in Figure 7.5A. The

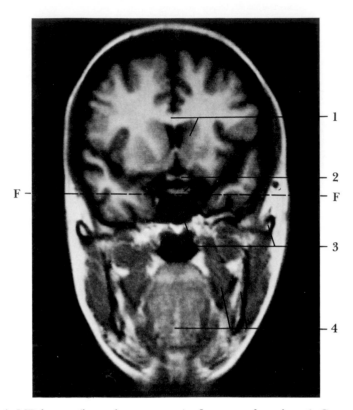

FIG. 7.4. MR image (inversion recovery) of a coronal section. *1*, Corpus callo-sum, caudate nucleus; *2*, optic nerve, pituitary gland between internal carotid arteries, lateral fissure; *3*, oropharynx, sphenoid air sinus, zygomatic arch; *4*, tongue, pterygoid muscle, mandible with masseter muscle. F-F plane of section of Figures 7.1 and 7.3B (Courtesy of General Electric, Medical Systems)

explanation for this is the slight downward tilt of the image. A normal axial MR image at the pituitary level, although slightly asymmetrical, demonstrates excellent anatomic detail (Fig. 7.6). The branches of the superficial temporal artery, the tendon of the superior oblique muscle, and the intracavernous internal carotid artery are all easily distinguished.

Cisterns   The *cisterns* around the brain stem, cerebellum, and diencephalon form an interconnected system of communicating spaces (Fig. 7.7); the cisterns are continuous not only with the subarachnoid space in the cerebral fissures and sulci but also with the subarach-noid space around the spinal cord. Several cisterns were seen in earlier illustrations, and others will be shown in subsequent chap-ters. The important *suprasellar* and *circummesencephalic* (ambient) cisterns occupy a pivotal position in the CSF flow from the poste-rior fossa, through the incisura of the tentorium, to the extensive

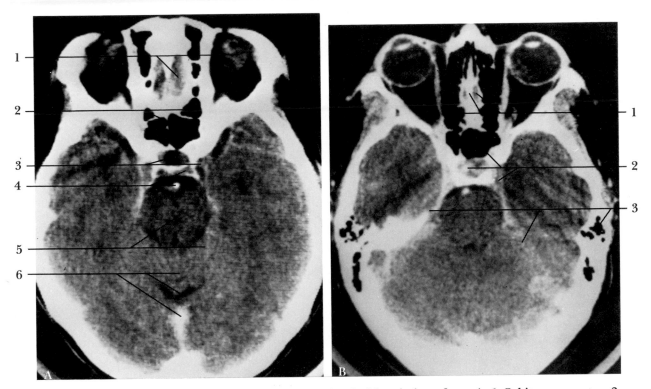

FIG. 7.5. CT images with contrast enhancement at the level of the pituitary fossa. **A.** *1,* Orbit, gyrus rectus; *2,* ethmoid air cells, sphenoid air sinus; *3,* cavernous sinus, pituitary gland around "empty sella"; *4,* basilar artery, dorsum sellae; *5,* tentorium, pons-midbrain transition; *6,* vermis, supracerebellar cistern, straight sinus. **B.** Image of a different, younger patient. *1,* Ethmoid air cells, crista galli, olfactory bulb; *2,* pituitary, sphenoid air sinus, cavernous sinus; *3,* fifth nerve, top of petrous pyramid, air cells in temporal bone.

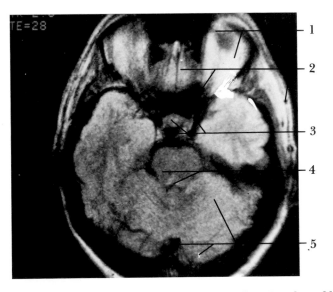

FIG. 7.6. Axial MR image (spin echo) at pituitary level. *1,* Tendon of left superior oblique muscle, orbital fat; *2,* gyrus rectus, sphenoid air sinus, branch of superficial temporal artery; *3,* dorsum sellae, pituitary, intracavernous internal carotid artery; *4,* pons, fourth ventricle, petrous pyramid; *5,* straight sinus near confluence, occipital lobe, cerebellar hemisphere.

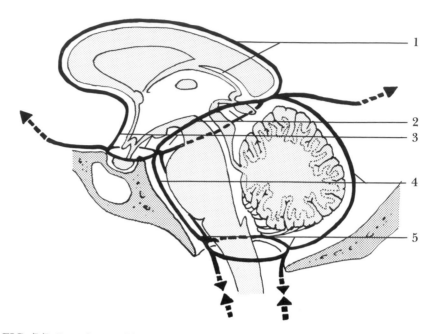

FIG. 7.7. Drawing to illustrate the interconnections of cisternal (subarachnoid space) spaces. *1*, Callosal cistern, cistern of velum interpositum; *2*, left ambient cistern, quadrigeminal cistern; *3*, cistern of the lamina terminalis, suprasellar cistern, interpeduncular cistern; *4*, pontine cistern, supracerebellar cistern; *5*, medullary cistern, cisterna magna.

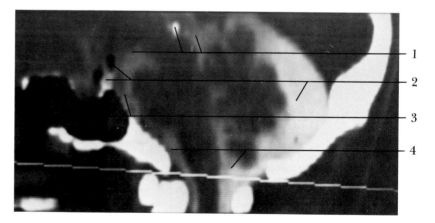

FIG. 7.8. CT cisternogram reformatted into midsagittal plane. *1*, Interpeduncular cistern, calcified pineal gland, quadrigeminal cistern; *2*, dorsum sellae, air in suprasellar cistern, supracerebellar cistern; *3*, sphenoid air sinus, basilar artery in pontine cistern; *4*, medullary cistern, cisterna magna. The white line shows that the lower level of the foramen magnum makes an angle with the infraorbitomeatal base plane (see Chapter 8).

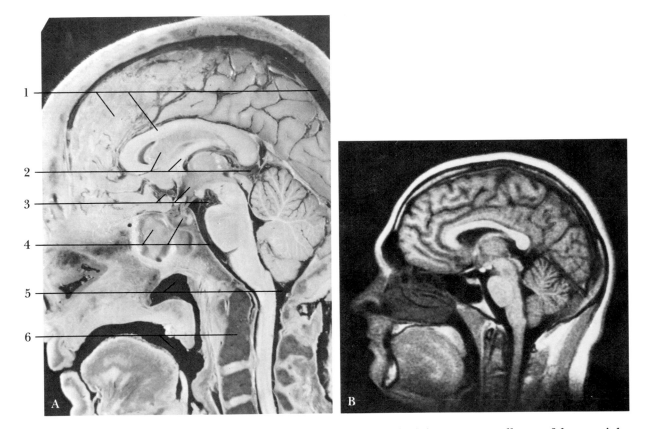

FIG. 7.9. Midsagittal images. **A.** Anatomic section. *1,* superior sagittal sinus, corpus callosum, falx over right frontal lobe; *2,* pineal in quadrigeminal cistern, fornix above interventricular foramen, septum; *3,* interpeduncular cistern, hypothalamus, anterior cerebral artery; *4,* basilar artery, pituitary gland, septum in sphenoid air sinus; *5,* cisterna magna, nasopharynx; *6,* C2 vertebra (axis), oral cavity. (Unsöld, R., Ostertag, C.B., De Groot, J., and Newton, T.H.: Computer Reformations of the Brain and Skull Base. Berlin, Heidelberg, New York, Springer-Verlag, 1982.) **B.** MR inversion recovery. The anatomic detail is remarkably clear. (Courtesy of General Electric, Medical Systems)

sites of CSF absorption in the supratentorial compartment. Other cisterns are identified in the legend of Figure 7.7. A representative, reformatted CT cisternogram is shown in Figure 7.8; a normal midsagittal anatomic section (Fig. 7.9) enables a comparison.

Because the anatomic relationships change so rapidly between the level of the suprasellar cistern (Fig. 6.3) and the level of the mid-pons (Fig. 7.3), this region is often examined with thinner cuts, e.g., 3-mm or even 1.5-mm thick, to avoid inaccurate interpretation due to volume-averaging.

Reformations

Another advantage of serial thin sections is that special computer programs allow the reformation (or reconstruction) of the available data into other planes with reasonable accuracy. A midsagittal image cannot be directly obtained with CT, while with the MR method sagittal and parasagittal structures are easily visualized (as seen earlier). A midsagittal view, e.g., by CT reformation through the sella region and posterior fossa, is sometimes required; it is very helpful in determining normal anatomy or the spatial relationships between normal structures or pathologic masses (compare Figs. 7.3 and 7.4 with 7.12). Similarly, coronal reformations may be used in such clinical situations. However,

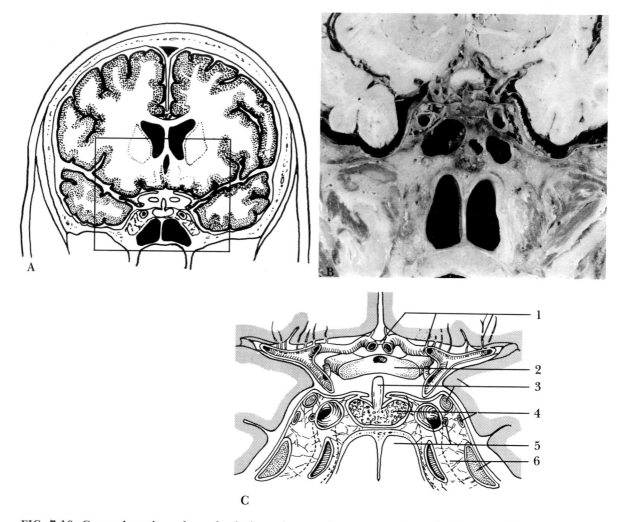

FIG. 7.10. Coronal sections through pituitary fossa and cavernous sinus. **A.** Drawing of coronal section through brain and skull base indicating the area enlarged in Figures 7.10B and 7.10C. Figure 7.10B is slightly asymmetrical; Figure 7.10C is not. **B.** Anatomic section. **C.** Illustration. *1,* Anterior communicating artery, medial and lateral lenticulostriate arteries off anterior cerebral artery and middle cerebral artery; *2,* optic chiasma with suprachiasmatic recess, intracranial internal carotid artery; *3,* pituitary stalk in suprasellar cistern, third nerve (oculomotor), uncus; *4,* pituitary gland within capsule, diaphragma sellae, fourth nerve (trochlear); *5,* sphenoid air sinus, intracavernous segment of internal carotid artery; sixth nerve (abducens); *6,* cavernous sinus, trigeminal ganglion.

unlike sagittal plane images with CT, coronal CT images may be obtained directly by hyperextension of the patient's neck. The pictures thus created are not in a true coronal plane with a 90° angle to the infraorbitomeatal base plane; rather, it slopes 100° to 120° backwards. Moreover, there are often metal artifacts from dental fillings that may degrade the image, and some patients do not tolerate such a maneuver. Therefore, one or more coronal reformations from a series of thin horizontal (axial) slices are sometimes preferred, although the reformatted image appears slightly poorer in quality (and costs more computer time).

Coronal sections through the normal sellar region are seen in Figure 7.10. Note the sequence of nerves in the lateral aspect of the cavernous sinus, in the twice-cut carotid; and in the spaces above and below the pituitary gland. It is an important area for the understanding of the anatomy and symptomatology of pituitary tumors, craniopharyngiomas, aneurysms, etc.

A dissection of the left cavernous sinus in three stages is shown in Figure 7.11; the IIIrd, IVth, first division of the Vth, and VIth cranial nerves are seen converging towards the supraorbital fissure. The (tortuous) intracavernous carotid and the optic nerve are identifiable. The abducens (VIth) nerve, entering the cavernous sinus from below, passes between the internal carotid artery and trigeminal ganglion; it is the nerve most often affected by intracavernous carotid dilatation.

Altered Anatomy

A CT cisternogram with reformations through the pituitary region is shown in Figure 7.12. The axial image shows an enlarged, partially empty sella. The midsagittal reformation, Figure 7.12A, illustrates the size of the sella; the infundibulum appears to end nowhere, but the axial image shows that the pituitary gland is compressed mainly to the left side of the sella. This finding is confirmed by the coronal reformation in Figure 7.12B. Note how the contrast is present in all cisterns, the fourth ventricle and aqueduct, and the third ventricle (Fig. 7.12A). The coronal reformation shows the unenhanced cavernous sinuses lateral to the sella; the cave of Meckel for the trigeminal ganglion contains contrast, which is a normal finding.

In Figure 7.13, a rounded mass is seen lying in the suprasellar cistern; the differential diagnosis included aneurysm, pituitary adenoma, and craniopharyngioma. Other scans and an angiogram made the diagnosis clear: a meningioma of the tuberculum sellae (another example of "look-alikes").

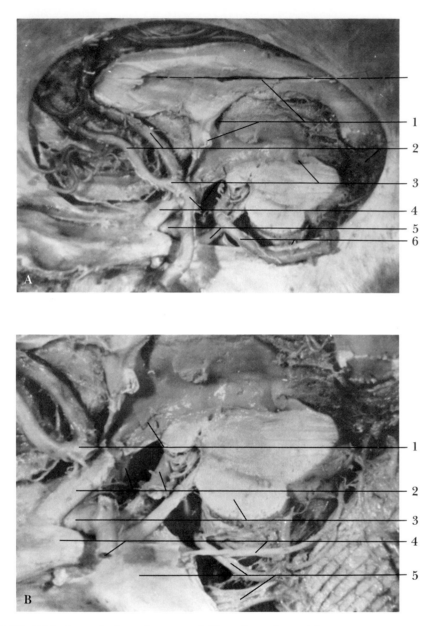

FIG. 7.11. Lateral view of stages of dissection of cranial nerves at cavernous sinus. **A.** The left hemisphere has been removed. The main arteries are viewed laterally, with the third ventricle and midbrain exposed. *1,* Interventricular foramen, anterior commissure, cut in corpus callosum and septum according to plane in Figure 4.2; *2,* left and right anterior cerebral artery, great cerebral vein; *3,* anterior communicating artery, suprasellar cistern, aqueduct; *4,* left optic nerve, left anterior cerebral artery, *5,* left internal carotid artery, third nerve; *6,* left posterior cerebral artery, free edge of tentorium. **B.** The tentorium has been removed so that four cranial nerves are seen in their intradural course. *1,* Anterior communicating artery, hypothalamus; *2,* left optic nerve, pituitary stalk, left posterior cerebral artery; *3,* internal carotid artery, cerebral peduncle; *4,* left anterior clinoid process, middle cerebral artery, fourth nerve; *5,* dura lateral to cavernous sinus, superior cerebellar artery, fifth nerve.

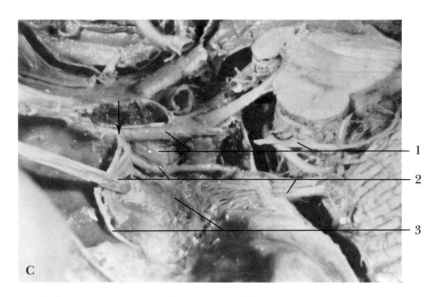

C. The left cavernous sinus has been exposed by removing the overlying dura. *1*, Intracavernous internal carotid artery, third nerve, proximal portion of fourth nerve; *2*, ophthalmic division of fifth (reflected) nerve; sixth nerve, main root of V; *3*, fourth nerve (reflected); fifth nerve ganglion. Note the convergence of nerves towards the superior orbital fissure *(arrow)*.

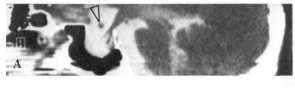

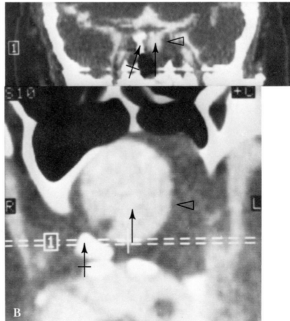

FIG. 7.12. Reformations of a series of thin CT sections with contrast in the cisterns. **A.** In the midsagittal reformation the basal cisterns are well filled; the pituitary fossa is enlarged and filled with contrast. Note the filling defect of the optic chiasma *(arrowhead)*; the posterior cerebral artery is seen near the interpeduncular cistern; hence the irregular contours in the lower part of these images. **B.** A coronal reformation; the corresponding axial plane is shown. Note the empty sella *(arrows)* with the pituitary pushed to the left side *(arrowheads)*. The dorsum sellae was averaged in *(crossed arrows)*.

Clinical Cases

CASE 12

An 18-year-old male clerk had increasingly complained of HAs for approximately the last year. When looking straight ahead, he also had difficulty seeing objects to one or the other side and would bump into objects or people not directly in front of him. He felt that he was not fully developed sexually and had no sexual interests. He had difficulty keeping warm in cold weather.

NEX: Incomplete bitemporal HAO. PR, 58; BP, 100/65. No secondary sexual characteristics.

What is the DDX? A CT scan was done (Fig. 7.14). Describe your findings. Can you explain the black line (or cross) in the sella on the axial cut? What is your DX?

(Discussion of Case 12 and additional illustrations on p. 210.)

CASE 13

A 43-year-old white man had complaints similar to those of the patient in Case 12: HA, bitemporal HAO, reduction in libido. However, he was normally developed sexually, had three children, and stated that he was happily married. On careful ques-

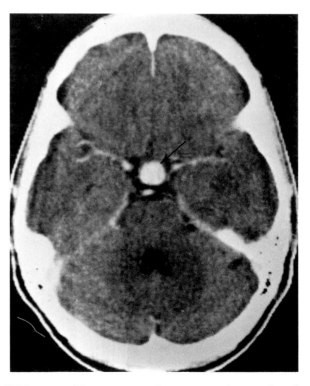

FIG. 7.13. CT image with contrast enhancement. A round, enhancing mass *(arrow)* is present in the suprasellar cistern.

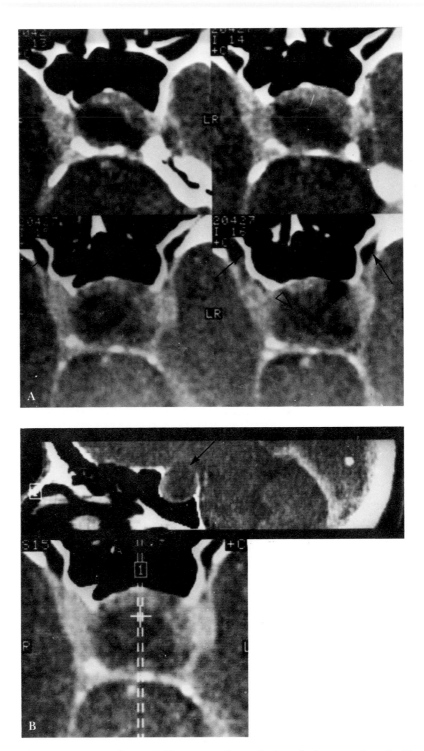

FIG. 7.14. Contrast-enhanced CT images through the pituitary region. **A.** Four axial sections, 1.5 mm apart, are seen through an enlarged sella; note the linear artifacts *(arrowheads)*, and the fat density in the superior orbital fissure *(arrows)*. **B.** A midsagittal reformation shows an enlarged pituitary *(arrow)* with a suprasellar extension and a bulging floor.

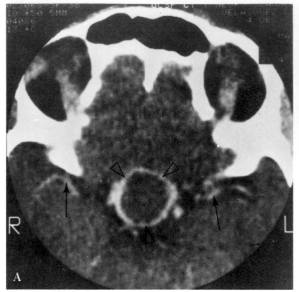

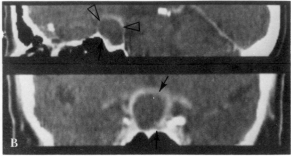

FIG. 7.15. Contrast-enhanced CT images through the suprasellar region. **A.** A large, round mass with enhancing rim *(arrowheads)* is seen between the middle cerebral arteries *(arrows)*. **B.** Midsagittal and coronal reformations. The location of the mass *(arrowheads)* is visualized more clearly within and above the enlarged sella; a small amount of pituitary tissue is still present *(arrows)*.

tioning, it became clear that his visual problems had become manifest *first,* his endocrinologic problems later.

A CT scan was done (Fig. 7.15A). A large, rounded, suprasellar mass was seen, containing an enhancing rim, central low density, and a suggestion of calcification on the R side (confirmed by CT measurement). On reformations (Fig. 7.15B) the sella appeared mildly enlarged; the mass seemed to have grown *down into* the sella, compressing the pituitary gland to the side.

What is your DDX? Would you do an angiogram? Why?

(Discussion of Case 13 and additional illustrations on p. 210.)

Questions

7a. Which cerebral lobes are present in Figure 7.3? In Figure 7.6?

7b. Figure 7.10B is an enlargement of Figure 7.4; why is the internal carotid artery visible twice in this axial slice?

7c. Name the lowermost gyrus of the frontal lobe (medially above the olfactory bulb and peduncle).

7d. What is the CT density of the fourth ventricle? Is it higher or lower than the pons?

7e. What structure and what space lie just *below* the pituitary gland? What structure and what space are just *above* the gland?

8. Lower Posterior Fossa (*Anatomic Slices G and H*)

Normal Anatomy

The first slice lies at the level of the infraorbitomeatal plane, so that the lower orbit and the external auditory meatus can be distinguished in Figure 8.1A. The two important areas at this level are (1) *posterior fossa* with *internal auditory meatus, pons, fourth ventricle,* and *cerebellum;* and (2) the *orbit* and *paranasal sinuses* (ethmoid cells, sphenoid air sinus, and, somewhat lower, the maxillary air sinus). This second area is discussed further in Chapter 9. The second slice lies at the level of the upper medulla and lower fourth ventricle. (Figs. 8.1B and 8.2).

The posterior fossa is bounded anterolaterally by the *petrous pyramid* (containing a labyrinth) on each side, as well as by the *clivus* (lateral to which the internal carotid arteries and the trigeminal ganglia are located; the posterior boundary is the occipital bone.

The anatomic compartments at this level can be seen in Figure 8.3, which is representative of a section at the infraorbitomeatal base plane, the orientation base plane for standard CT sections. Note that the anterior cranial fossa is no longer visible, and the middle fossa contains only the lower portions of the *temporal lobes.* The *sphenoid air sinus* and *clivus* lie below and behind the pituitary fossa, and close to the intrapetrosal portion of the *internal carotid.* Lateral to these large vessels the *trigeminal ganglia* can be seen with their forward extensions (at this level), the maxillary divisions.

The details of this area are seen in Figure 8.4. Note the *pons; cranial nerves* V, VI, VII, and VIII; the *flocculus* in the cerebellopontine angle; the *fourth ventricle* with choroid plexus and lateral

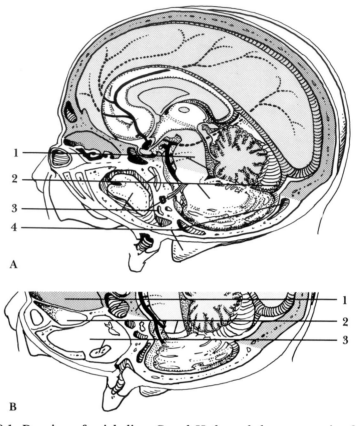

FIG. 8.1. Drawing of axial slices G and H through lower posterior fossa. **A.** Upper slice (G). *1,* Pons, fourth ventricle, basilar artery; *2,* occipital sinus, cerebellar white matter, carotid canal within petrous pyramid; *3,* bony labyrinth, nerves VII and VIII in internal auditory meatus, lowermost part of temporal lobe; *4,* transverse sinus, mastoid process. **B.** Lower slice (H). *1,* Nasal cavity, sphenoid air sinus, clivus; *2,* maxillary air sinus, left vertebral artery, medulla; *3,* temporal fossa, mandible, sigmoid sinus.

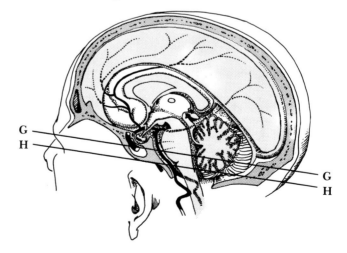

FIG. 8.2. Drawing of midsagittal structures and spaces illustrating levels of slices G and H.

apertures; the cerebellar *tonsils; vermis;* and lateral hemispheres. There is an arachnoid granulation in the *sigmoid sinus;* this common finding confirms that such granulations are present in all sinuses and large veins, not merely in the superior sagittal sinus (such arachnoid structures are thought to give rise to meningio-

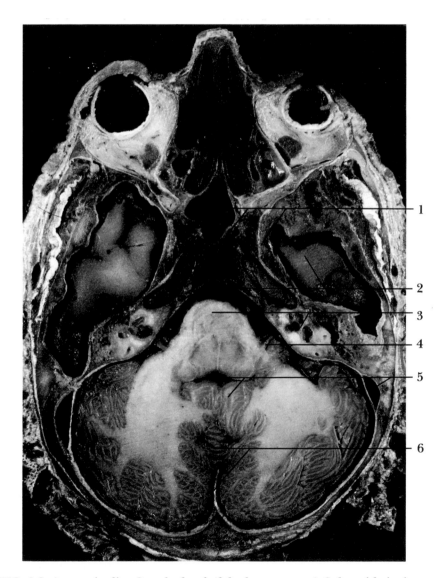

FIG. 8.3. Anatomic slice G at the level of the lower pons. *1,* Sphenoid air sinus, clivus, trigeminal ganglion; *2,* basilar artery, internal carotid, lowermost temporal lobe; *3,* pons, VIth nerve, labyrinth in petrous pyramid; *4,* VIIth nerve, flocculus; *5,* fourth ventricle, cerebellar tonsil, sigmoid sinus; *6,* inferior vermis, falx cerebelli.

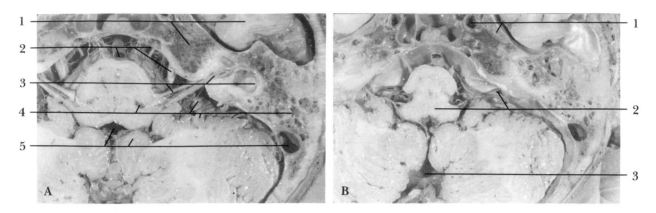

FIG. 8.4. Anatomic axial section through the lower posterior fossa. **A.** Section through cerebello-pontine angle region. *1*, Petrous pyramid, temporal lobe; *2*, abducens nerve, trigeminal nerve, basilar artery; *3*, semicircular canal, internal auditory meatus, facial nerve; *4*, air cells, flocculus, pia of pontomedullary junction; *5*, sigmoid sinus, tonsil, ventricle. (Unsöld, R., Ostertag, C.B., De Groot, J., Newton, T.H.: Computer Reformations of the Brain and Skull Base. Berlin, Heidelberg, New York, Springer-Verlag, 1982.) **B.** Section through the medulla. *1*, Internal carotid artery, trigeminal ganglion; *2*, medulla, IXth nerve entering jugular foramen; *3*, foramen magnum.

mas). Arachnoid trabeculae can be seen in the region of the *basilar artery*, as well as the VIth (abducens) nerves on both sides, across from the *inferior petrosal sinuses*. The *petrous pyramid* contains the *internal auditory meatus*, with the VIIth (facial) and VIIIth (vestibulocochlear) nerves, the cochlea (cross-cut), and the *semicircular canals* (two are seen); more laterally, the *mastoid air cells* are beginning to show.

The next lower slice lies parallel to and below the infraorbitomeatal base plane and represents usually the second cut made in a routine series of CT scans through the head and brain (Figs. 8.1B, 8.2, 8.4B, and 1.3). The posterior fossa contains the *medulla*, with lowermost cranial nerves, *fourth ventricle* with cerebellar *tonsils*, portions of the *sigmoid sinus*, and the *internal jugular bulb*. The *mastoid air* cells are more clearly seen, as are the *internal carotid foramina* in the base of the skull. The *glenoid fossae*, where the articulations with the mandible occur, are seen more anteriorly and laterally; sometimes portions of the *external auditory meatus* may be seen. The various deep muscles of the face lie behind the *nasal cavity* with its septum, and the *maxillary air sinuses*.

Cranial Nerves

The *cranial nerves of the posterior fossa*, important anatomic and functional structures, are seen in their intracranial course in Figure 8.5. Many nerves course for a considerable distance through the various cisterns (ambient, lateral pontine, cerebellopontine, medullary); others have a shorter transcisternal extent. The *IVth* cranial nerve (trochlear) courses around the midbrain, partially under the free edge of the tentorium; the *Vth* nerve (trigeminal) *ganglion* lies in a dura pocket (cave of Meckel), from which the main root connects to the lateral pons. The *VIth* nerve (abducens) is not shown; it exits ventrally, courses briefly through the (pre)pontine cistern, then pierces the dura to enter the cavernous sinus. The *VIIth* and *VIIIth* nerves (facial with intermedius, vestibulocochlear) pass into the internal auditory meatus within the petrous pyramid, to innervate the labyrinthine sense

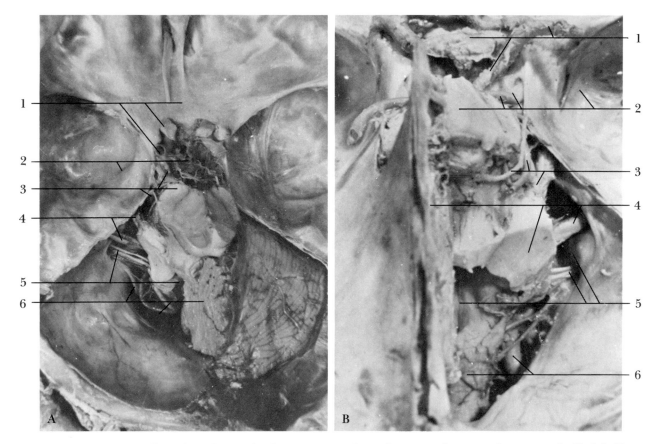

FIG. 8.5. Anatomic dissection of posterior fossa contents. **A.** Brain stem and nerves after removal of left half of cerebellum (oblique view). *1*, Planum sphenoidale, optic nerve, internal carotid; *2*, suprasellar cistern with contents, temporal fossa; *3*, midbrain, IIIrd nerve, IVth nerve; *4*, Vth nerve, VIIth and VIIIth nerves entering internal auditory meatus; *5*, fourth ventricle, IXth and Xth nerves passing through jugular foramen; *6*, vermis, posterior inferior cerebellar artery, XIth nerve emerging from cisterna magna. **B.** Posterior view of brain stem and cranial nerves; right half of cerebellum and tentorium removed. *1*, chiasma, large right posterior communicating artery, middle cerebral artery; *2*, midbrain, posterior cerebral artery IIIrd nerve, temporal fossa; *3*, IVth nerve, superior cerebellar artery, Vth nerve; *4*, "seam" of tentorium and falx, middle cerebellar peduncle, VIIIth nerve; *5*, floor of fourth ventricle, IXth and Xth nerves, cerebellopontine angle; *6*, medulla, right vertebral artery.

organs (VIII) or pass through the skull base (VII). Cranial *nerves IX, X, and XI* (glossopharyngeal, vagus, accessory) all pass through the jugular foramen, together with the major draining venous channels. The *XIIth* nerve (hypoglossal) is not visible; it exits from the ventral medulla as a series of rootlets.

Coronal Sections

Some of the *main arteries of the posterior fossa* are partly seen in Figure 8.5. Included are the vertebral, posterior inferior cerebellar, and the superior cerebellar arteries; the basilar artery and anterior inferior cerebellar artery are not shown. All arteries are seen in their relationship to the brain stem in Figure 8.6. Note the posterior cerebral artery above the tentorium; the three pairs of cerebellar arteries are seen in a rather normal orientation below the tentorium. There is considerable variation in the origin of the cerebellar arteries from the vertebral and basilar arteries. An oblique coronal section shows the (intracranial) basilar artery between the (intrapetrosal) internal carotid arteries (Fig. 8.7). The *middle ear cavities* with ossicles are visible, as well as the cartilaginous portions of the *Eustachian tubes*.

Three additional sequential coronal sections show the anatomic relationships of the posterior fossa elements to the supra-

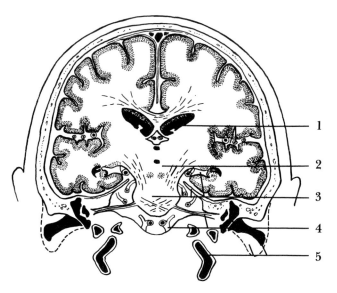

FIG. 8.6. Drawing of coronal section through brain stem. *1,* Lateral ventricle, lateral fissure; *2,* midbrain, cerebral peduncle, posterior cerebral artery; *3,* pons, superior cerebellar artery, tentorium, temporal horn; *4,* vertebral artery with posterior inferior cerebellar artery, internal auditory meatus with nerves, middle ear cavity; *5,* internal carotid, mastoid process, external auditory meatus.

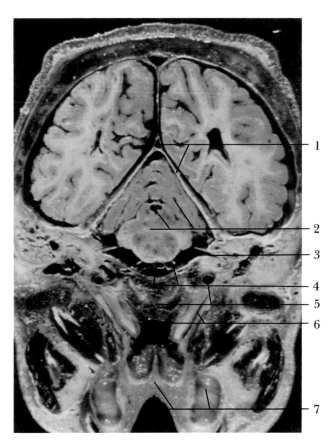

FIG. 8.7. Oblique coronal anatomic section through posterior fossa. *1*, Straight sinus, tentorium, occipital horn; *2*, pons, fourth ventricle, cerebellum; *3*, internal auditory meatus with VIIIth nerve, middle ear cavity; *4*, basilar artery, VIth nerve; *5*, clivus, internal carotid; *6*, nasopharynx, Eustachian tube; *7*, oral cavity, palate, maxillary air sinus.

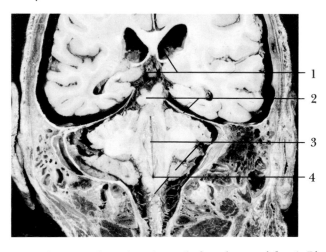

FIG. 8.8. Anatomic coronal section through fourth ventricle. *1*, Pineal gland, great vein, right lateral ventricle; *2*, colliculi, tentorium, temporal horn; *3*, fourth ventricle, cerebellum; *4*, obex, medulla, XIth nerve.

tentorial structures and spaces, the tentorium, and the skull base (Figs. 8.8, 8.9, and 8.10). The most anterior one (Fig. 8.8) cuts across the *foramen magnum,* floor of the *rhomboid fossa* (fourth ventricle), *quadrigeminal plate,* pineal region, atria, and inferior horns. Figure 8.9 is a section through the *posterior fourth ventricle* and (enlarged) posterior horns; several *dural sinuses* are shown. The plane of Figure 8.10 cuts through the *cerebellum* behind the fourth ventricle and shows its vermis and tonsils. Note the varying slope of the tentorium in these three coronal sections, and how high its apex reaches between the occipital lobes (coronal CT cisternograms are presented in Chapter 10).

Images through the lower posterior fossa are shown in Figure 8.11A (CT image) and Figure 8.11B (MR image); they are from two different persons. The planes of section and therefore the anatomic relationships are almost identical; a direct comparison between the two neurodiagnostic methods is possible. The streak-artifacts seen in the CT image are absent in the MR image. On the other hand, the details of bony structures are better seen on CT images. Figure 8.12A is a bone window CT section at approximately the same level as Figures 8.11A and B. The air cells in the mastoid process, middle ear ossicles, and the foramina all appear with great clarity. An even more detailed image is shown in Figure 8.12B; the ossicles, scutum (bony ridge for attachment of the tympanic membrane), the elements of the bony labyrinth, are all seen quite clearly. Such special bone window images are

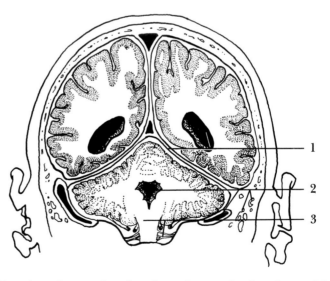

FIG. 8.9. Drawing of coronal section through posterior fourth ventricle. *1,* Tentorium, atrium-posterior horn transition; *2,* fourth ventricle, sigmoid sinus, mastoid air cells; *3,* medulla, XIIth nerve, posterior inferior cerebellar artery.

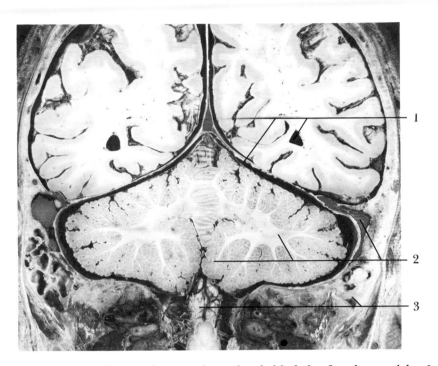

FIG. 8.10. Normal coronal anatomic section behind the fourth ventricle. *1*, Straight sinus, tentorium, posterior horn; *2,* tonsil, dentate nucleus, sigmoid sinus; *3,* medulla, mastoid process.

useful in determining not only normal bone anatomy, but also bone erosion by tumors, bone thickening with other tumors, or fractures. In the posterior fossa and elsewhere in the head or in the vertebral region, such pathologic bone changes can be readily seen with CT, but not (yet) in similar detail with the MR method.

Another comparison between images obtained in various ways is made in Figure 8.13. In Figure 8.13A the normal CT image does not provide detailed anatomic information; Figure 8.13B is an MR image of the same region (on a slightly different plane), providing excellent detail of the posterior fossa without streak-artifacts. However, the combination of a CT cisternogram and a high window setting results in an image of a satisfactory quality for most cases (Fig. 8.13C). In fact, posterior fossa lesions are often examined with the latter method, if necessary.

Altered Anatomy: An axial CT image with a wide window setting through the base of the skull, slightly lower than the image seen in Figure 8.11A, is shown in Figure 8.14. The pathology is at first rather subtle, until (and unless) the obligatory comparison is made be-

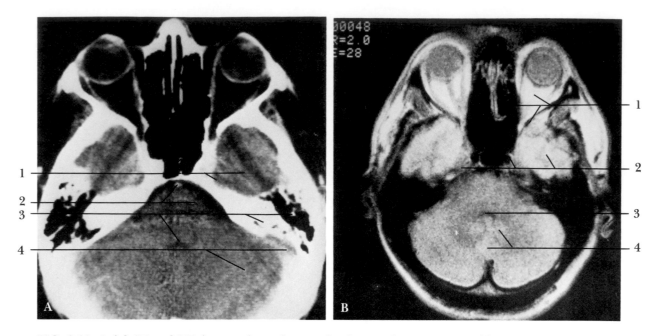

FIG. 8.11. Axial CT and MR images through posterior fossa and petrous pyramids. **A.** CT image without contrast enhancement. *1*, Temporal lobe with artifact, low density of Vth nerve ganglion, sphenoid air sinus; *2*, pons with artifact, calcified basilar artery in pontine cistern; *3*, auditory ossicles, petrous pyramid, fourth ventricle; *4*, sigmoid sinus, cerebellum. **B.** MR image (spin echo). *1*, Ethmoid air cells, sphenoid bone, orbit; *2*, trigeminal ganglion, internal carotid artery, temporal lobe; *3*, fourth ventricle, petrous pyramid; *4*, vermis, tonsil.

tween the left and right side. (A soft tissue window setting at this level and higher showed a mass in the left middle fossa.) The bone window image shows obliteration of the left foramen ovale and changes in the surrounding skull base. This was due to a slowly growing, rare tumor, a schwannoma of the maxillary nerve.

Another patient had increasingly complained of hoarseness, and later of general malaise, headache, and dizziness. Two axial images through the lower posterior fossa show a bone-eroding mass extending from the level of the jugular foramen (Figs. 8.15A and B). The lower extent of the tumor is defined by a direct coronal CT image, Figure 8.15 (compare Figs. 8.6 and 8.7). The differential diagnosis was neurofibroma (note first complaints) or a chemodectoma, a rare, highly vascular tumor of this region. Angiography was done to make the final diagnosis.

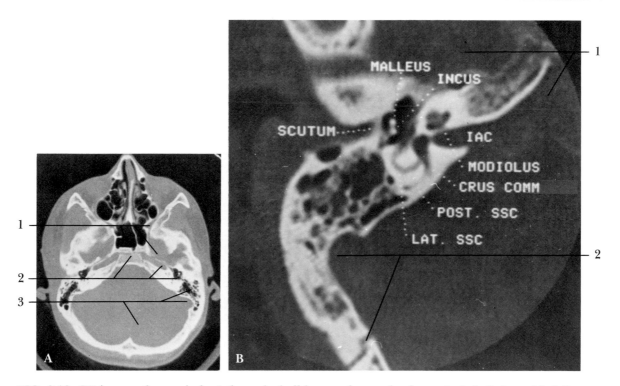

FIG. 8.12. CT images (bone window) through skull base and posterior fossa. **A.** *1,* Inferior orbital fissure, temporal lobe, sphenoid air sinus; *2,* left middle ear, internal carotid artery, clivus; *3,* sigmoid air sinus, air cells, posterior fossa. **B.** Details of right petrous pyramid. *1,* middle fossa, region of the pons; *2,* sigmoid sinus, lambdoid suture.

A female patient with gradual hearing loss in one ear of some 2 years duration had more recently noticed asymmetry of her face and increasing weakness of the face muscles on the same side. There was occasional double vision. Figure 8.16 shows CT images obtained by injecting a small amount of air via LP into the posterior fossa of the patient, who is then placed in a lateral recumbent position with the diseased side up. The CT air cisternogram in Figure 8.16B shows an enlarged internal auditory meatus and a tumor mass projecting into the cerebellopontine angle cistern. This picture is typical of an VIIIth nerve Schwannoma. For comparison, a normal CT air cisternogram is shown in Figure 8.16A.

Two examples of posterior fossa tumors, examined by the MR method, are shown in Figures 8.17 and 8.18. The posterior fossa and fourth ventricle are distorted in both cases. In Figure 8.17 a mass in the anterior portion of the cerebellopontine angle cistern was found to be an epidermoid tumor. Note the difference between the two spin echoes. The other tumor (Fig. 8.18) in a 7-year-old girl caused obstructive hydrocephalus by blocking the

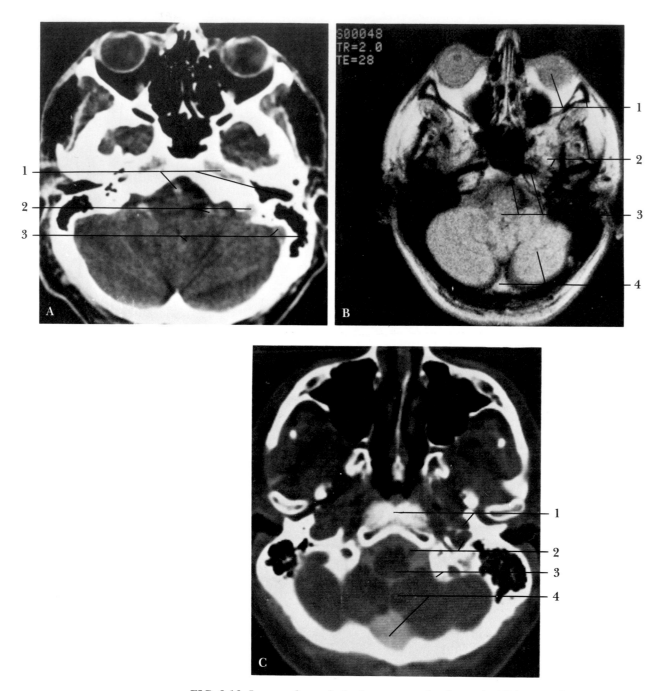

FIG. 8.13. Images through the lower posterior fossa. **A.** CT image with contrast enhancement. *1*, Internal carotid artery, external auditory meatus, basilar artery; *2*, jugular bulb, choroid plexus near flocculus; *3*, mastoid air cells, sigmoid sinus, fourth ventricle. **B.** MR image (spin echo). *1*, Maxillary air sinus, globe, zygomatic bone; *2*, foramen ovale, foramen spinosum with artery, coronoid process of mandible; *3*, medulla, basilar artery, internal carotid artery; *4*, internal occipital protuberance, cerebellar hemisphere. **C.** Normal CT cisternogram. *1*, clivus, carotid canal; *2*, vertebral artery, part of jugular foramen; *3*, medulla, jugular tubercle; *4*, tonsil, cisterna magna (part).

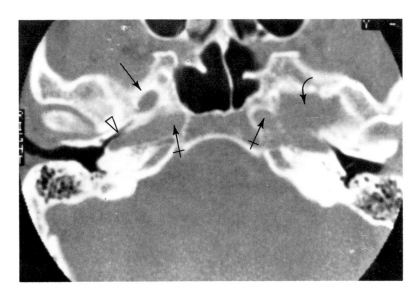

FIG. 8.14. Axial CT image (bone window) through base of skull. On the normal right side, the Eustachian tube is seen *(arrowhead)* and the foramen ovale *(arrow)*. The carotid canal is seen on both sides *(crossed arrows)*. On the abnormal side the foramen ovale has been destroyed by an osteoclastic Schwannoma *(curved arrow)*.

outflow foramina; its location (vermis) is typical for a medulloblastoma, a malignant radiosensitive tumor of childhood, that often seeds along the CSF pathways at the skull base or into the spinal dural sac.

Clinical Cases

CASE 14

A 12-year-old school girl began over the last several months to develop a tendency to trip and fall when playing with other children. More recently she had difficulty walking. She had a tendency to vomit shortly after waking up, and she complained of headache "in the neck."

NEX: Ataxic gait; FTN and HTS tests very poor; dysmetria. DTRs lively, and bilateral plantar extensor responses. Bilateral PE, spontaneous nystagmus. No neck stiffness. Plain skull films did not show any abnormality. CBC wnl.

What is your DDX at this stage? Would you consider asking for a high myelogram or a CT cisternal study? Why? Why not?
A CT scan was done (Fig. 8.19). What are your findings in the supratentorial compartment? In the posterior fossa? How can you explain all this? Now what is your DX?

(Discussion of Case 14 on p. 211.)

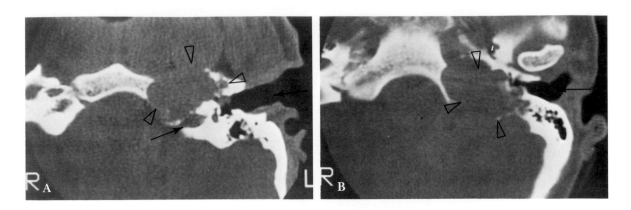

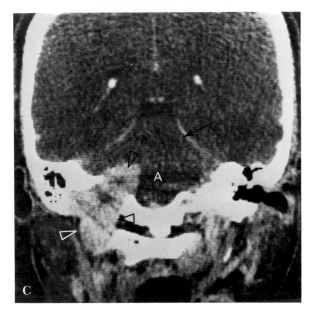

FIG. 8.15. CT images through the base of skull and posterior fossa. **A.** Axial image. A large destructive mass is seen *(arrowheads)* below the internal and external auditory meatuses *(arrows)*. **B.** In a lower axial section, the mass is seen to occupy the region of the jugular foramen *(arrowheads)*; the external auditory meatus is still seen *(arrow)* posterior to the mandibular process. **C.** Direct coronal CT image through posterior fossa. The mass seen in Figure 8.15A is seen to extend below the skull base *(arrowheads)*. The tentorium *(arrow)* and a dark streak-artifact *(A.)* are noted.

CASE 15   A 41-year-old man complained of double vision, tremor in the hands, deteriorating eyesight, and increasing weakness and unsteadiness in the extremities. The S/S had been present for at least 6 months. He also complained of "creeping" feelings in his fingers.

NEX: Poorly muscled man with weakness in all four extremities. Ataxic gait of the "wide-based" variety. Bilateral weakness of

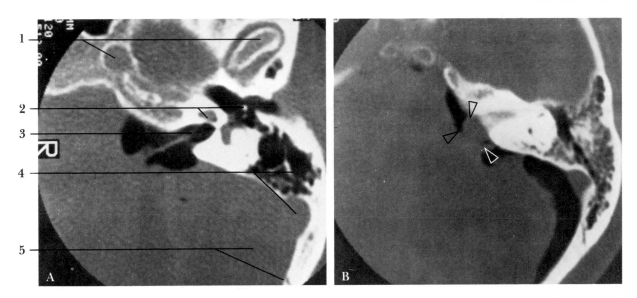

FIG. 8.16. Axial CT images taken with the patient lying on left side. Air was injected earlier to fill the lateral posterior fossa. **A.** Normal image. *1,* Mandible, carotid canal; *2,* ear ossicles, cochlea; *3,* branching of VIIIth nerve within internal auditory meatus, air in cerebellopontine angle; *4,* mastoid air cells, sigmoid sinus; *5,* cerebellum, lambdoid suture. (Courtesy of Dr. D. LaMasters). **B.** In the abnormal image, a small mass *(arrowheads)* is seen within the cerebellopontine angle; the internal auditory meatus is widened.

the lateral rectus muscle. Difficulty on L or R lateral gaze. FTN and HTS tests grossly abnormal. Increased DTRs. There was considerable loss of all sensory modalities in the extremities.

Lab data: BP, 130/95; CBC: WBC, wnl; RBC, 4.5M. CXR: wnl.

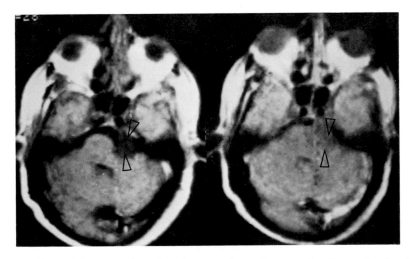

FIG. 8.17. Axial MR (spin echo) images through posterior fossa. In the left image (first echo), a low-signal area *(arrowheads)* was shown to be an epidermoid tumor; in the right image a longer echo delay produces a higher signal intensity in the tumor, indicative of its long T2.

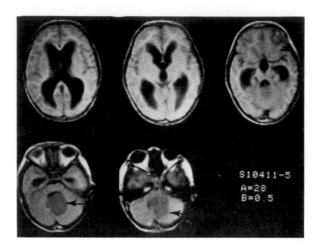

FIG. 8.18. Serial axial MR (spin echo) images of a 7-year-old male patient. A low-signal mass is seen in the vermis region of the cerebellum *(arrows)*; the fourth ventricle is compressed and blocked, resulting in hydrocephalus.

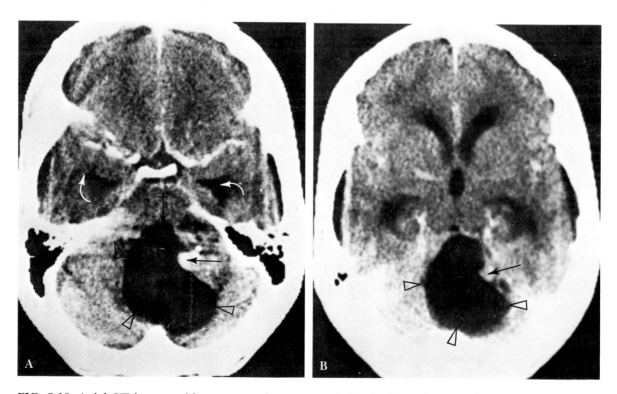

FIG. 8.19. Axial CT images with contrast enhancement. **A.** In the lower image, a large low-density mass *(arrowheads)* is seen containing a high-density mural nodule *(arrow)*; the fourth ventricle is compressed *(crossed arrow)* and the temporal horns are enlarged *(curved arrows)*. **B.** The same mass *(arrowheads)* and nodule *(arrow)* are protruding high under the tentorium; the ventricles are enlarged.

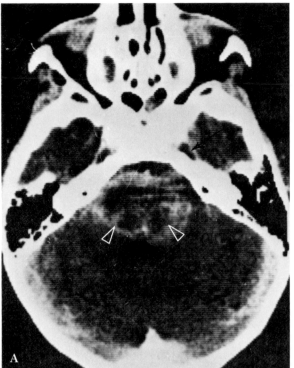

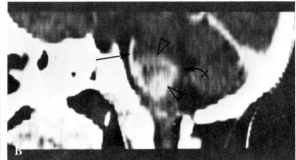

FIG. 8.20. CT images with contrast enhancement. **A.** In the axial image, a large mass *(arrowheads)* with irregular densities and streak-artifacts occupies the region of the pons; the pontine cistern is mildly compressed. The low density of the left trigeminal ganglion is shown *(arrow)*. **B.** In a midsagittal reformation, the same mass *(arrowheads)* is seen between the basilar artery *(arrow)* and fourth ventricle *(crossed arrow)*; the pontine cistern is still visible.

What is your DDX? Which neuroradiologic diagnostic procedures would you require? For what purpose?

A CT scan was done (Fig. 8.20). What are your findings, i.e., what anatomically visible changes are seen and what changes in CT density? Where? Now what is your DX?

(Discussion of Case 15 and additional illustration on p. 213.)

Questions

8a. Viewed along an infraorbitomeatal plane series of cuts, which cerebral lobe is the lowest?

8b. What lies between the orbits?

8c. Which structures course within the internal auditory meatus?

8d. What is the best way (using neuroradiologic methods) to obtain an image of the internal auditory meatus and labyrinth?

8e. Which components of the venous drainage system of the brain are visible in Figure 8.9?

8f. Which of the paranasal sinuses are seen in Figure 8.1? Which on Figure 8.7?

8g. Explain how suppurative mastoiditis can result in septicemia (see Fig. 8.4A or 8.6).

8h. How can the lambdoid suture best be visualized on CT, e.g., to differentiate it from a bone fracture?

9. Orbit

Orbital Axial Plane

The usual CT planes (infraorbitomeatal, direct or reformatted coronal, and reformatted sagittal) have proved unsatisfactory for an adequate CT examination of orbital contents, because the axis of each orbit itself is different from any of the standard planes. Therefore an axial plane has been adopted that has a 10° to 15° negative angulation from the standard axial CT plane; thus it courses parallel to the optic nerves (Figs. 9.1 and 9.2).

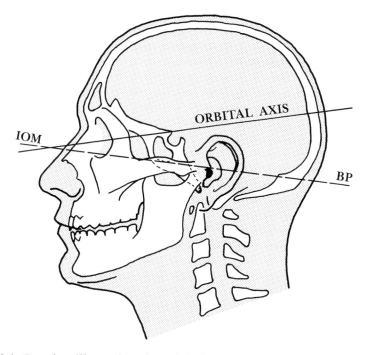

FIG. 9.1. Drawing illustrating the axial plane used in scanning of the orbit.

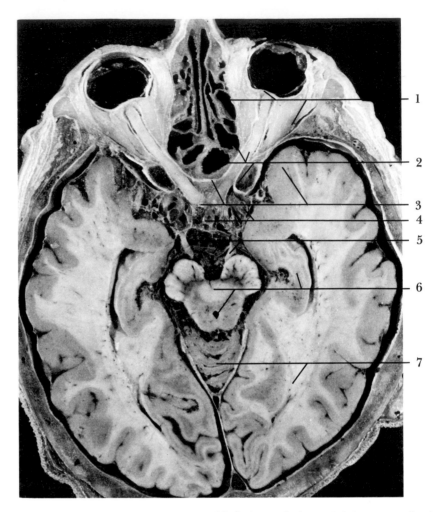

FIG. 9.2. Anatomic section through orbital plane of Figure 9.1 (upper surface). *1*, Ethmoid air sinus, right optic papilla, lateral rectus; *2*, sphenoid air sinus, optic nerve in orbital apex, anterior clinoid process; *3*, optic chiasma, tuberculum sellae, temporal lobe; *4*, infundibulum, internal carotid artery; *5*, suprasellar cistern, basilar artery, right IIIrd nerve; *6*, midbrain, aqueduct, hippocampus medial to temporal horn; *7*, cerebellum, optic radiation. (Unsöld, R., Ostertag, C.B., De Groot, J., and Newton, T.H.: Computer Reformations of the Brain and Skull Base. Berlin, Heidelberg, New York, Springer-Verlag, 1982.)

Normal Anatomy

The orbits are separated by the *paranasal sinuses* medially; the orbital axes make an angle of about 80° with each other (Fig. 9.2). The *optic chiasma* lies in the middle cranial fossa, just in front of the *infundibulum* and between the intracranial internal carotid arteries. The *temporal poles* extend forward, lateral to the *orbital apex* and *anterior clinoid processes*. The *midbrain* is found behind the *suprasellar cistern* and in front of the *upper cerebellum*.

The *optic nerves* within the orbit have a sinuous course, thus permitting rotatory movement of the eyeball with different gaze directions. To determine if one nerve is different in size than the other (e.g., in optic glioma or sheath meningioma), special orbital planes and reformations are necessary from a series of thin sections parallel to the orbital axial plane (Fig. 9.3).

Reformations

These orbital reformations allow for direct comparison between left and right eyes by showing the nerves, muscles, and tendons in each eye in a more comparable way, and at right angles to the plane of section (Figs. 9.4A and B). The optic nerve can neither be seen nor evaluated in its entirety in any single oblique sagittal or axial plane because of its sinuosity.

An oblique-sagittal reformatted cut along the optic nerve, oblique to the midsagittal plane of the head, is seen in Figure 9.4. In the anatomic section, the nerve is considerably more curved, probably because of fixation in downward gaze. In the CT image the muscles, nerves, and vessels can be easily identified because these structures have a different CT-density than the very low density of the (intraorbital) fat.

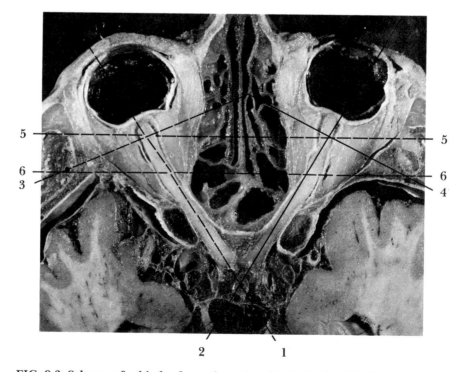

FIG. 9.3. Scheme of orbital reformations. *1* and *2:* Orbital axial planes; *3* and *4:* orbital coronal planes; *5* and *6:* true coronal planes.

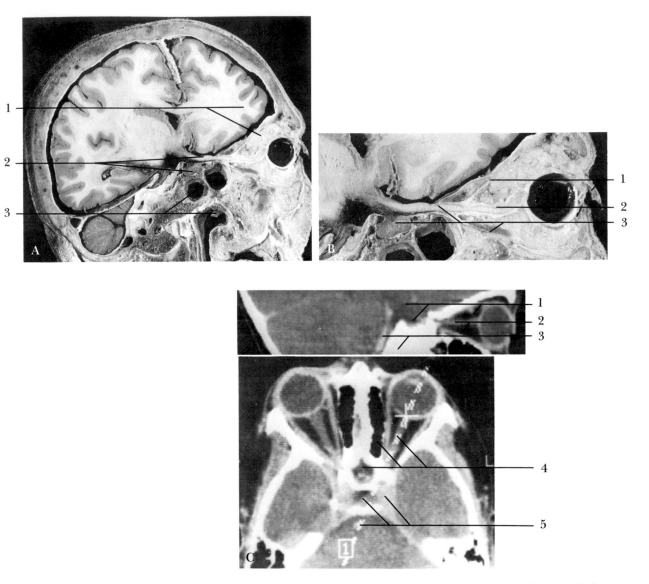

FIG. 9.4. Left orbital axial plane. **A.** Anatomic orientation. *1*, Left frontal lobe, orbit; *2*, optic chiasma, pituitary gland within sella turcica; *3*, nasopharynx, sphenoid air sinus. **B.** Orbital details of Figure 9.4.A. *1*, Superior rectus, globe, eyelid; *2*, optic nerve; *3*, pituitary gland, nerve in optic canal, inferior rectus. **C.** Corresponding CT image. *1*, Suprasellar cistern, sella, superior orbital vein under superior rectus; *2*, optic nerve, inferior rectus; *3*, basilar artery, clivus; *4*, sphenoid air sinus, ethmoid air sinus, plane of left optic nerve; *5*, basilar artery, sella, left cavernous sinus.

The relationships of the orbital structures to the adjacent anatomic areas are demonstrated in detail in the anatomic sections in Figure 9.5. *Eyeballs, extraocular muscles* and the *optic nerve* with its *meningeal sheaths* are seen intraorbitally, while the course of the optic nerves through the *optic canal* into the *optic chiasma* is

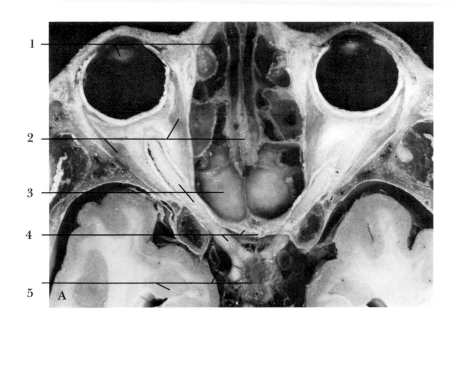

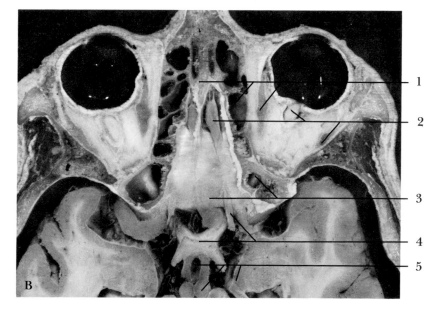

FIG. 9.5. Anatomic images in a plane close to the orbital scanning plane. **A.** Planum sphenoidale from below. *1,* Ethmoid air cell, sclera, lens of right eye; *2,* nasal septum, medial rectus, lateral rectus; *3,* planum, optic nerve in orbital apex; *4,* tuberculum sellae, intracranial optic nerve, anterior clinoid process; *5,* infundibulum, interior carotid artery, amygdala in front of inferior horn. **B.** Planum sphenoidale from above. *1,* Crista galli, ethmoid air cell, medial rectus; *2,* right olfactory bulb, optic nerve, lateral rectus; *3,* planum, bony canal for optic nerve in aerated sphenoid bone; *4,* chiasma, suprasellar cistern, olfactory peduncle; *5,* infundibular recess, mamillary body, uncus.

clearly demonstrated. The *air sinuses* separating the orbits are situated below the *planum sphenoidale, olfactory structures,* and *frontal lobes.* The temporal lobes, *suprasellar cistern,* and *cavernous sinuses* (not shown in Fig. 9.5) lie behind the orbits (see Fig. 9.2). Pathologic changes in intraorbital structures may thus affect the spaces and structures around the orbits (including the maxillary air sinuses).

Coronal sections through the orbits show these relationships clearly (Fig. 9.6). The anatomic sections resemble much-used CT reformations that permit direct comparison between the two orbits and intraorbital structures (Fig. 9.7). An upward-angulated axial plane demonstrates how the optic canal courses in a different direction than the ipsilateral superior orbital fissure (Fig. 9.8). The cranial nerves within the cavernous sinus are seen lateral to the carotids and pituitary gland.

In Figure 9.9 the direction of the optic canals is shown even more clearly, between the anterior clinoid processes laterally, and the tuberculum sellae medially. This anatomic section lies along the orbital axis; it is clear why this is the preferred plane for the CT examination of the orbit (compare with Fig. 9.8). Moreover, this plane demonstrates much of the visual pathways, from the retina, chiasma, and geniculate bodies to the occipital lobe (see also Fig. 9.2). The intraorbital anatomy can be demonstrated in

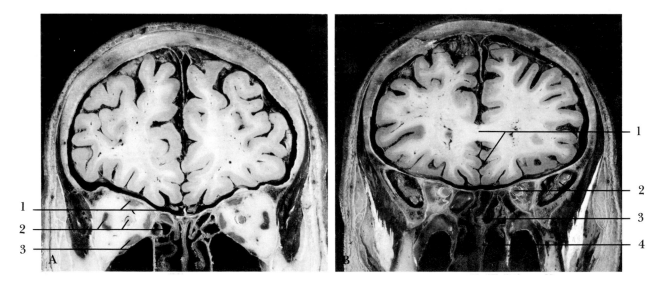

FIG. 9.6. Anatomic coronal sections. **A.** Section is just behind the globe. *1,* Olfactory stalk, superior orbital vein, superior rectus-levator complex; *2,* ethmoid air cell, optic nerve, lateral rectus; *3,* inferior rectus, maxillary air sinus. **B.** Section is close to the orbital apex. *1,* Corpus callosum (genu), interhemispheric fissure; *2,* optic nerve in orbital apex, temporal pole; *3,* sphenoid air sinus, ethmoid air cell; *4,* nasal septum, maxillary air sinus.

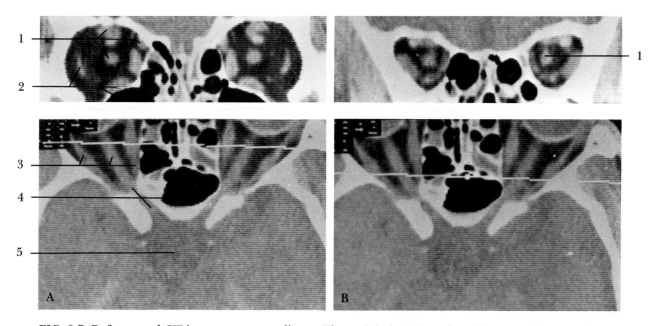

FIG. 9.7. Reformatted CT images corresponding to Figure 9.6. **A.** *1,* Superior oblique, optic nerve, levator palpebrae; *2,* inferior rectus, maxillary air sinus, lateral rectus; *3,* medial rectus, optic nerve, lateral rectus; *4,* sphenoid air sinus, optic canal; *5,* suprasellar cistern below and behind optic chiasma. **B.** *1,* The optic nerve is seen within a ring of muscles and vessels.

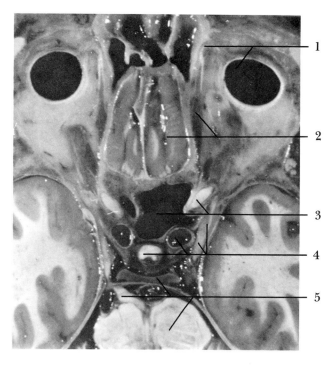

FIG. 9.8. Anatomic section (axial plane with upward angulation). *1,* Trochlea, left globe; *2,* left lower frontal lobe, superior oblique; *3,* sphenoid air sinus, optic nerve, and ophthalmic artery; *4,* pituitary gland, internal carotid artery (siphon), IIIrd and IVth nerves; *5,* right third nerve, dorsum sellae, midbrain.

axial MR images (Figs. 9.10 and 9.11). Optic nerves, extraocular muscles, bony elements, and pituitary fossa all can be identified readily in this 7-mm-thick section (Fig. 9.10).

Altered Anatomy

Figure 9.11 demonstrates the advantages of using different TE parameters: in Figure 9.11A the intraorbital and intraocular structures are seen, in a lower plane than in Figure 9.10 (same patient). The longer echo delay demonstrates the presence of a mass in the right eye with a short T1 and a short T2 (Fig. 9.11B). Note how the signal-to-noise ratio has decreased in Figure 9.11B. The MR imaging method of visualizing in and around the orbit (and elsewhere in the body) is beginning to equal that of CT; in

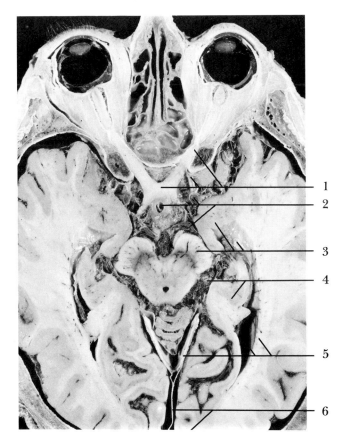

FIG. 9.9. Anatomic section (lower surface) through plane of Figure 9.1 to show the visual pathways (in part). *1,* Optic chiasma, olfactory peduncle, left optic nerve in canal; *2,* infundibular recess, left internal carotid artery, posterior cerebral artery; *3,* midbrain, amygdala, temporal horn; *4,* medial geniculate body, hippocampus; *5,* tentorium, temporal horn, optic radiation; *6,* posterior falx, occipital lobe. (Unsöld, R., Ostertag, C.B., De Groot, J., and Newton, T.H.: Computer Reformations of the Brain and Skull Base. Berlin, Heidelberg, New York, Springer-Verlag, 1982.)

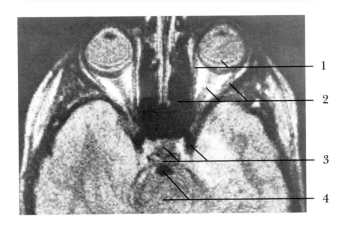

FIG. 9.10. Normal axial MR image (second echo) through the orbit. *1,* Medial rectus, eye motion artifact; *2,* ethmoid air cells, optic nerve, lateral rectus; *3,* dorsum sellae, pituitary, left anterior clinoid process and internal carotid artery; *4,* midbrain, large basilar artery. There is a high-intensity abnormality in the left temporal lobe.

addition, the various display modes of MR imaging may soon give considerable insight not only into the anatomy of the orbit, but also into the chemical aspects of physiologic and pathologic changes.

A mildly abnormal anatomic image is seen in Figure 9.12; the mass within the sphenoid air sinus is a retention cyst of a mucous gland; it may, rarely, obtain aggressive properties by growing and destroying the surrounding structures (mucocele). In the patient seen in Figure 9.12 the retention cyst was an inci-

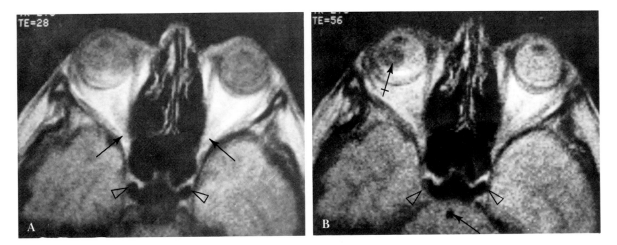

FIG. 9.11. MR images through the orbit. **A.** First echo. Internal carotid arteries *(arrowheads)* are clearly seen within the cavernous sinus; the superior orbital fissures contain fat *(arrows)*. **B.** Second echo. The internal carotid arteries *(arrowheads)* and basilar artery *(arrow)* are seen. An intraocular tumor (melanoma) with a short T2 is seen in the right globe *(crossed arrow)*.

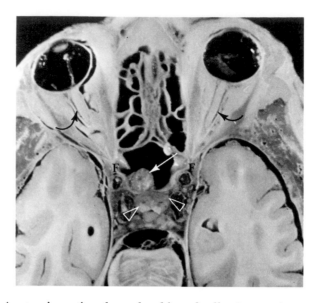

FIG. 9.12. Anatomic section through orbit and sella. A retention cyst is seen in the sphenoid sinus *(arrow)* in front of the pituitary gland *(arrowheads)*; the meningeal sleeves *(curved arrows)* around the optic nerves are clearly seen as well as the extra-ocular muscles. *F* = superior orbital fissure.

dental finding. Note also the cone of muscles in the orbit, the right orbital canal "protruding" into the sphenoid air sinus (compare Fig. 9.5B), and the relationship between cavernous sinus and superior orbital fissure.

Figure 9.13 demonstrates a CT image in the orbital-axial plane of a tumor involving the optic sheath; this meningioma typically contains calcification, causes proptosis, and leads to ipsilateral blindness.

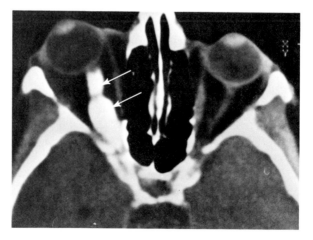

FIG. 9.13. CT image with contrast enhancement. In the right orbit a high-density mass *(arrows)* is seen grown into the optic nerve; this is a meningioma. There is minimal dilation of the orbital apex.

Clinical Cases

CASE 16

During a pre-employment physical exam the following was noted in a 29-year-old woman: mild exophthalmos (right more than left), infrequency of winking, weakness of convergence. Also, there was a fast tremor of the hands and generalized weakness of the trunk and extremity muscles. A preliminary diagnosis was made on the basis of endocrine tests, and the woman was referred to a neuro-ophthalmologist. After examining her, he requested a CT scan with reformations (Figs. 9.14 and 9.15).

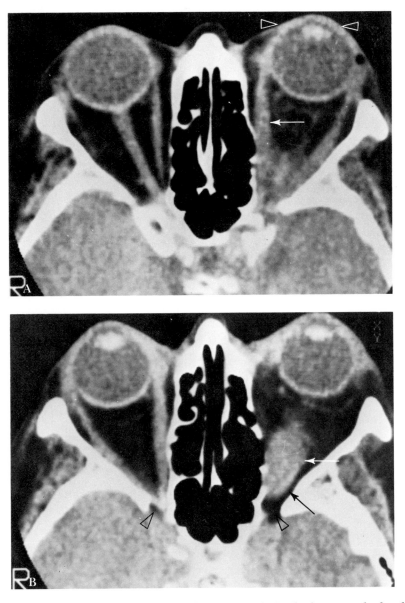

FIG. 9.14. CT images with contrast enhancement. **A.** In the image at the level of the clinoids, a slightly enlarged medial rectus *(arrow)* is seen in the proptotic left orbit *(arrowheads)*. **B.** In the image at a lower level, an enlarged inferior rectus is seen *(arrows)*; note the normal fat in the superior orbital fissures *(arrowheads)*.

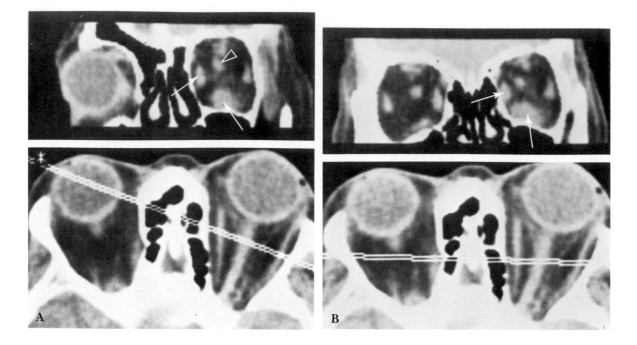

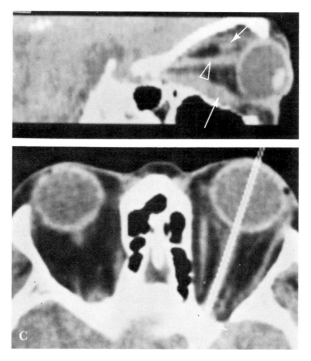

FIG. 9.15. Computer reformations through the orbits of Figure 9.14. **A.** In the orbital coronal reformation the enlarged inferior and medial rectus muscles *(arrows)* are seen in relation to the optic nerve *(arrowhead)*. **B.** True coronal reformation, comparing the enlarged muscles *(arrows)* with the normal ones in the right orbit. **C.** The orbital-axial reformation shows the enlarged left inferior rectus *(arrow)* below the optic nerve *(arrowhead)*; the superior orbital vein *(crossed arrow)* is seen below the normal superior rectus.

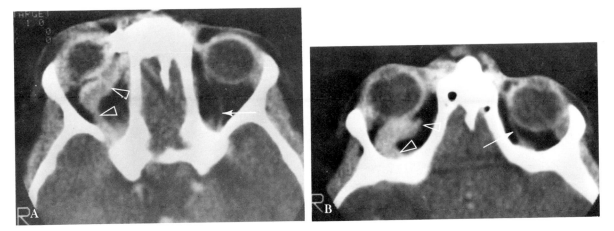

FIG. 9.16. Contrast-enhanced CT images through the orbits. **A.** An enlarged right superior orbital vein *(arrowheads)* is seen in comparison with the normal left one *(arrow)*. **B.** A similar finding is seen.

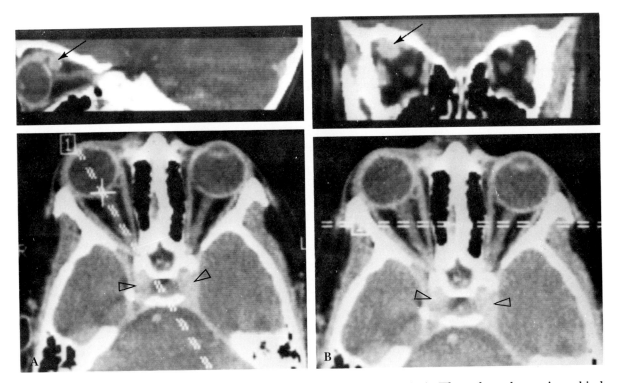

FIG. 9.17. Orbital-axial reformations through right orbit of Figure 9.16. **A.** The enlarged superior orbital vein *(arrow)* is seen in cross section; the cavernous sinuses *(arrowheads)* are equal in size. Note the lower density within the enlarged vein in Figures 9.16 and 9.17A, representing the fluid center of the vessel. **B.** This figure permits direct comparison between the diameter of the left and right superior orbital veins.

What are your findings on the scans?
What is your DDX? What is your DX?

(Discussion of Case 16 on p. 214.)

CASE 17   An 18-year-old female had had a severe superficial nasal infection (she suffered from chronic facial acne); she had fever and
general malaise and stayed in bed. One morning she woke up
with a swollen right eyelid, intraocular pain, and headache. Se-
verely ill, she was hospitalized; fundoscopy showed engorged
veins. A CT scan with reformation was done (Figs. 9.16 and 9.17).
    What are your findings? What was the pathophysiologic
process? What is your DX? Administration of antibiotics helped
to reverse the course of this potentially life-threatening series of
pathologic events.

(Discussion of Case 17 on p. 214.)

Questions   9a. What is the rationale for adopting an orbital CT plane that is
different from the standard infraorbitomeatal CT plane?
Why are so many reformations done routinely in neuro-oph-
thalmologic CT examinations?

9b. What would be the best way (using CT) to compare the caliber of one optic nerve with the other?

9c. The orbital veins are in communication with both superficial
facial veins and deep cranial sinuses. Why is that significant?

9d. The ophthalmic artery has extensive anastomoses with
branches of the external carotid artery. Why is that potentially (and practically) significant?

9e. In cases of carotid/cavernous (CC) communications (e.g.,
traumatic CC-fistula), what would be clearly abnormal in the
orbital CT?

9f. If a normal person is looking to the left, what would be the
position of the optic papilla in the right eye? Would it be
more lateral (temporal) than in the neutral position, or more
medial (nasal)?

9g. How could you demonstrate with CT methods the continuity
of the optic sheath with the intracranial subarachnoid space
in normal subjects?

10. Craniovertebral Junction

Normal
Anatomy

OSSEOUS
STRUCTURES

The craniovertebral junction is a complex transition zone that contains the structures adjacent to the foramen magnum, both in a cranial and a cervical direction.

The bony structures of this region include the *occiput, atlas or C1 vertebra,* and *axis or C2 vertebra* (Figs. 10.1 and 10.2). Several openings exist in the posterior skull base that permit entry or exit of vessels, nerves, and neuraxis (Fig. 10.2A); such foramina can be easily demonstrated on CT images (bone window) (Fig. 10.2B). The occipital condyles, atlas, and axis together form a complex of articulations, so that flexion, backward extension, and rotation of the head are mainly effected in the craniovertebral junction region.

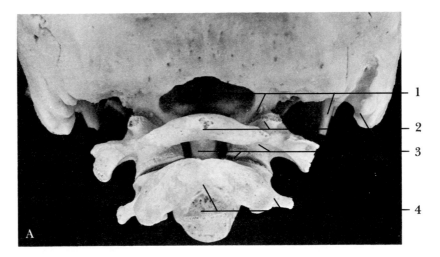

FIG. 10.1. Bony elements of craniovertebral junction. **A.** Posterior view. *1,* Foramen magnum, occipital condyle, styloid process; *2,* posterior arch of atlas, groove for vertebral artery, mastoid process; *3,* odontoid process, atlanto-axial joint, lateral mass of C1; *4,* body of C2 (posterior aspect), spinous process, transverse process. *(Fig. 10.1B is on p. 140.)*

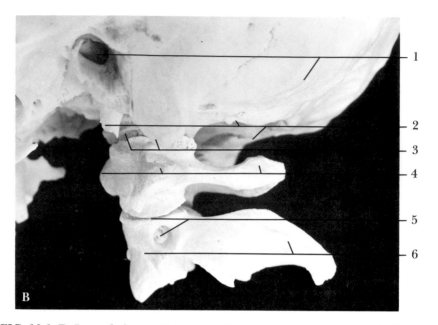

FIG. 10.1. **B.** Lateral view. *1*, External auditory meatus, occiput; *2*, styloid process, rims of foramen magnum; *3*, atlanto-occipital joint space, mastoid process; *4*, anterior arch, lateral mass, posterior arch of C1; *5*, atlanto-axial joint, foramen transversarium; *6*, body, spinous process of C2.

NEURAL
ELEMENTS

The neural elements of the craniovertebral junction consist of the *medulla,* lower *cerebellum,* and *upper cervical cord,* and the lower *cranial* and upper *cervical spinal nerves.* Two stages of a dissection of the dorsal aspects of the craniovertebral junction are shown in Figure 10.3. The nerve roots of *cranial nerves* VIII through XII and *spinal nerves* C1 and C2 are seen, coursing mostly laterally or lateroventrally to the neuraxis; the sensory roots of the C2 nerves enter dorsolaterally. Figure 10.3B shows, in addition, a number of arachnoid trabeculae and small vessels, rarely seen on CT. The region of the craniovertebral junction is associated with the *two vertebral arteries* that supply the vital centers in the brain stem, together with their continuation, the *basilar artery.* The main venous drainage *(jugular veins* and paraspinous *venous plexus)* from the skull likewise occurs in the region of the craniovertebral junction.

Sagittal and parasagittal sections through the craniovertebral junction show the anatomic relationships around the foramen magnum, especially with respect to the lower pole of the *cerebellar tonsils* (Fig. 10.4); normally, the tonsil should not extend below the plane connecting the lower edges of *clivus* and *occiput.* This plane makes a slight angle with the infraorbitomeatal plane (see

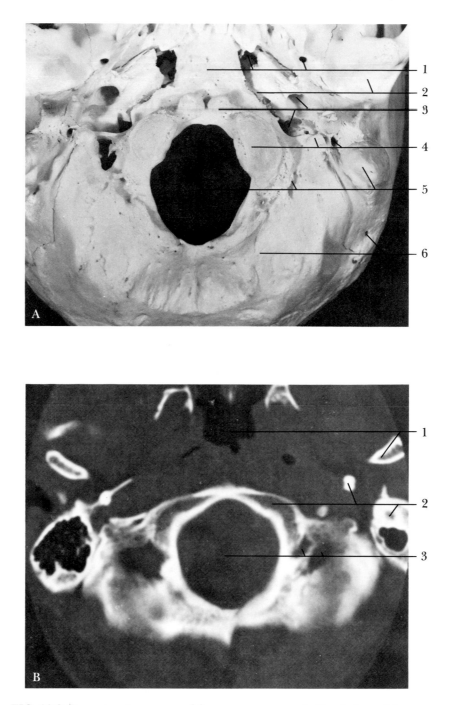

FIG. 10.2. Bony structures around foramen magnum. **A.** Basal view of the posterior skull base. *1*, Clivus, foramen lacerum, foramen spinosum; *2*, petro-occipital suture, glenoid fossa; *3*, mamillary process, jugular foramen, carotid canal; *4*, condyle, styloid process, stylomastoid foramen; *5*, foramen magnum, emissary foramen, mastoid process; *6*, occiput, emissary foramen. **B.** CT image, bone window. *1*, Nasopharynx, mandible; *2*, condyle, styloid process, mastoid process; *3*, foramen magnum, posterior condylar foramen (emissary), space below occiput (caused by thinness of slice).

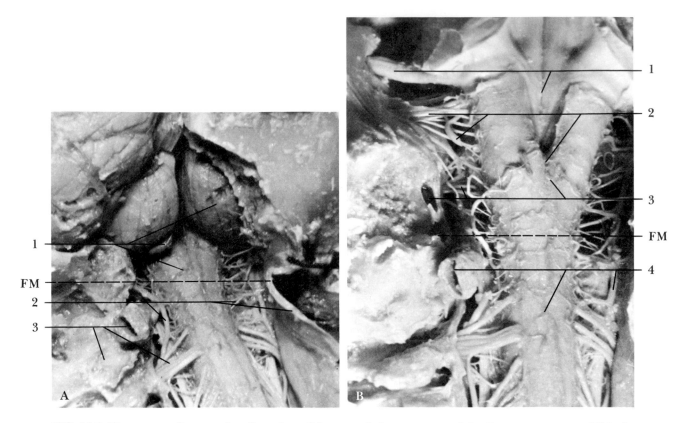

FIG. 10.3. Two stages of a posterior dissection of the neural elements around the foramen magnum *(FM)*. **A.** *1*, Posterior inferior cerebellar artery, closed medulla, cerebellar tonsil; *2*, rootlets of C1 nerve, cut edge of dura, left spinal accessory; *3*, vertebral artery, rootlets of C2 nerve, lateral mass of atlas. **B.** *1*, VIIIth nerve, floor of fourth ventricle; *2*, rootlets of vagus, branch of posterior inferior cerebellar artery, obex; *3*, emissary foramen, rootlets of hypoglossus, closed medulla; *4*, vertebral artery, C2 cord segment, right spinal accessory.

also Fig. 7.8). If the tonsil protrudes clearly below this inferior rim of the foramen magnum, the differential diagnosis should include *tonsillar herniation* ("coning") due to an intracranial mass, or congenital herniation of tonsils (the Chiari malformation); very rarely, the tonsils protrude below the foramen magnum as a normal anatomic variation.

CORONAL SECTIONS   Coronal sections demonstrate the elements of the region of the craniovertebral junction quite well: the articular facets of the *atlanto-occipital* joint slope medially downward, while the facets of the *atlanto-axial* articulation slope medially upward (Figs. 10.5A and 10.6). The facet joints not only contain cartilage that can be mildly compressed, but they are somewhat convex in several directions; thus the various movements of the head on the neck are made possible. Head movements are limited only by soft tissue mass, and especially the ligaments. An anatomic coronal section through the neuraxis of the craniovertebral junction region and cervical cord correlates with a similar MR image (Figs. 10.5B and C). The size of medulla and cord can thus be evaluated directly. Hyperextension of the head in a patient may be used in obtaining *direct coronal* CT images (Fig. 10.6; see also Fig. 1.2). Sometimes a direct coronal CT image cannot be obtained, e.g., the patient will not or cannot tolerate the necessary hyperextension, or, in more anterior areas, the dental fillings cause degrading artifacts in the image. Moreover, such images do not conform to the anatomic, true coronal plane seen in Figure 10.5, which can then be obtained by *reformatting* an image at a 90° angle from the infraorbitomeatal plane (Fig. 10.7).

The *lower cranial* and *upper cervical nerves,* including the *spinal accessory nerves,* can best be demonstrated in CT cisternograms (Figure 10.6C). The *vertebral arteries* enter the dura at the level of the C1 rootlets; the *posterior inferior cerebellar arteries,* usually

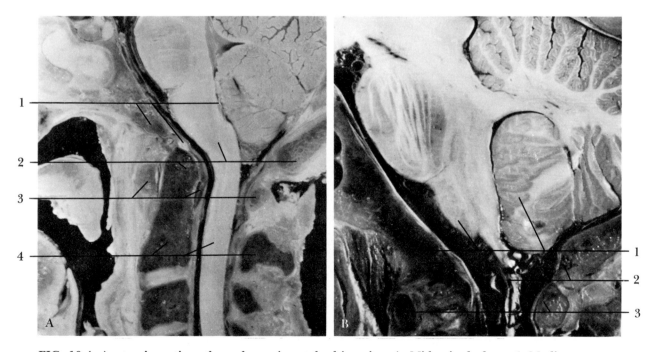

FIG. 10.4. Anatomic sections through craniovertebral junction. **A.** Midsagittal plane. *1,* Median aperture with choroid plexus, os odontoidum, clivus; *2,* occiput, closed medulla, dens; *3,* posterior arch of C1, transverse ligament, anterior arch; *4,* posterior elements of C2, spinal chord, body of C2. **B.** Parasagittal plane. *1,* Clivus, inferior olive, tonsil; *2,* lower end of medulla, occiput; *3,* anterior arch, posterior arch of C1.

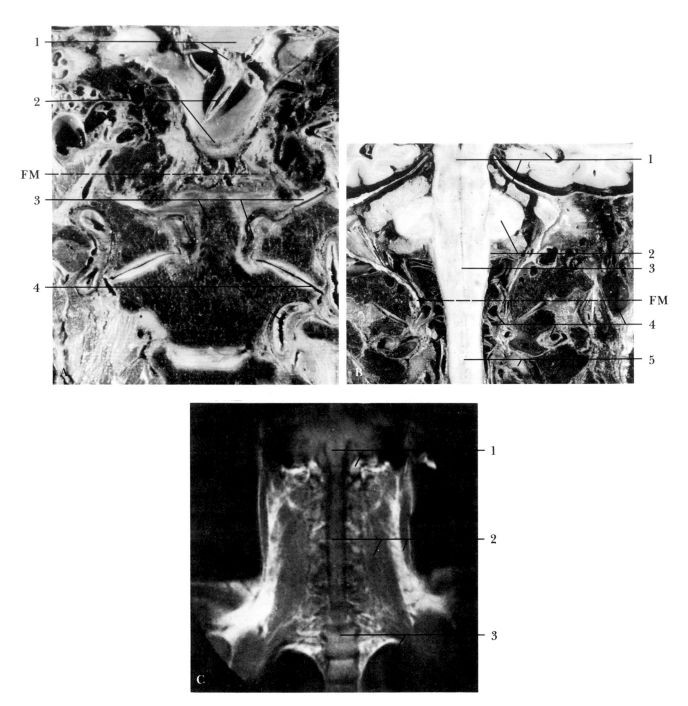

FIG. 10.5. Coronal sections through craniovertebral junction (FM, level of foramen magnum). **A.** *1*, Pons, basilar artery; *2*, left vertebral artery, clivus; *3*, atlanto-occipital joint, transverse ligament, dens; *4*, atlanto-axial joint, vertebral artery, body of C2. **B.** *1*, Midbrain, tentorium, hippocampus near inferior horn; *2*, rootlets of vagus, middle cerebellar peduncle, sigmoid sinus; *3*, medulla, hypoglossal rootlets stretched over posterior inferior cerebellar artery; *4*, rootlets of C1, intradural vertebral artery, vertebral artery, mastoid process; *5*, C2 segment of cord, dorsal root ganglion, lateral mass of C2. **C.** MR (inversion recovery) image. *1*, Medulla, jugular tubercle, mastoid process; *2*, cord, deep neck muscles, sternocleidomastoid muscle; *3*, T1 vertebral body, lung. (Courtesy of General Electric, Medical Systems)

branches of the vertebral arteries, are identifiable on CT images (Fig. 10.7).

Axial CT sections with normal window settings in the region of the craniovertebral junction are often not entirely satisfactory, in part due to the general volume-averaging effect, and more importantly due to streak-artifacts, caused by the marked differences in CT density of the various structures here (Fig. 10.8A). Figure 10.8B represents an image with a wide window (different subject), showing excellent detail of the skull base. Computed tomography studies at this level (or at any spinal level) are often improved by injection of a contrast agent into the subarachnoid space via a lumbar or C1/C2 puncture. Metrizamide, a water-solu-

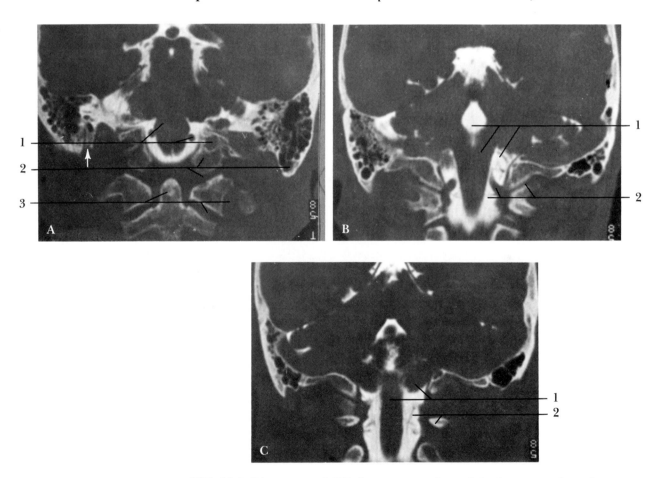

FIG. 10.6. Direct coronal CT cisternograms through brain stem and craniovertebral junction. **A.** Most anterior section. *1*, Jugular foramen, vertebral artery, medulla; *2*, mastoid process, atlanto-occipital joint, condyle; *3*, canal for vertebral artery, atlanto-axial joint, dens. Note facial canal *(arrow)*. **B.** *1*, Fourth ventricle, medulla, rootlets of vagus; *2*, rootlets of C1, vertebral artery, atlanto-occipital joint. **C.** *1*, Medulla-cord transition and level of foramen magnum, tonsil; *2*, spinal accessory, lateral elements of C1.

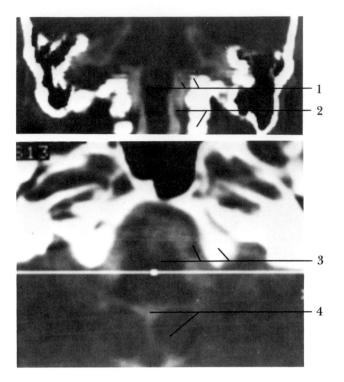

FIG.10.7. Coronal reformation from C2 axial cisternogram (compare with Figure 10.6B). *1*, medulla, posterior inferior cerebellar artery, jugular tubercle; *2*, vertebral artery, lateral element of C2, mastoid process; *3*, medulla, left vertebral artery, jugular tubercle; *4*, fourth ventricle, tonsil.

ble, nonionizing agent, is commonly used. The resulting images can then be shown with different window settings (soft tissues or bone), so that a comprehensive visualization of the region is achieved (Figs. 10.6, 10.7, 10.8, and 10.9).

A normal series of CT cisternograms of the lowermost posterior fossa is seen in Figure 10.9, with an anatomic section for comparison (Fig. 10.9C; see also Chapter 8). Note how the major vessels and bony landmarks stand out; the contours of the brain stem are much better seen in this figure than in Fig. 10.8. There are few artifacts seen in Figure 10.9. Computed tomography cisternograms are best used to determine the site of a lesion: intra-axial (within the neuraxis) or extra-axial (in the vessels, subarachnoid space, meninges, or bone).

Magnetic Resonance Images

A series of normal MR images through the lower posterior fossa and foramen magnum is seen in Figures 10.10A and B (different patients) and 10.11A and B (same patient). There are no streak-artifacts, and the various tissues can be easily distinguished. As elsewhere in the body, the rate of blood flow in the larger vessels can be judged by the signal intensity, from fast-flowing (no signal) to occlusion (high-intensity signal). The high contrast between normal flowing blood and the vascular wall precisely defines the luminal contours, and indicates the presence of atherosclerotic narrowing. Intimal abnormalities may be detected without contrast agents that may sometimes obliterate a small lesion.

The muscles at the anterior skull base and in the neck stand out and are quite easily identifiable (Figs. 10.10A and 10.11A). The configuration of the medulla, cerebellum, and tonsils is clearly seen (compare with Fig. 10.8). However, when the second echo is obtained, the muscles lose signal intensity, and the definition of the cerebello-medullary complex is much decreased, due to the increased signal of the CSF (long T2; Fig. 10.11B).

The axial levels just below the foramen magnum are shown in Figures 10.12 and 10.13, both in anatomic sections and in CT images. Spinal nerve C1 lies just above the *atlas,* whereas the *rootlets* for *C2* are found at the level of the atlas and just below, forming a spinal nerve passing between *atlas* and *axis* (see also Fig. 10.3). In anatomic sections, the relationship between the *odontoid* process of C2 or dens, the *transverse ligament,* and the anterior arch of *C1* are clearly seen (Figs. 10.4A and 10.12A). Slightly lower, the sloping *atlanto-axial facets* are seen cut obliquely in axial sec-

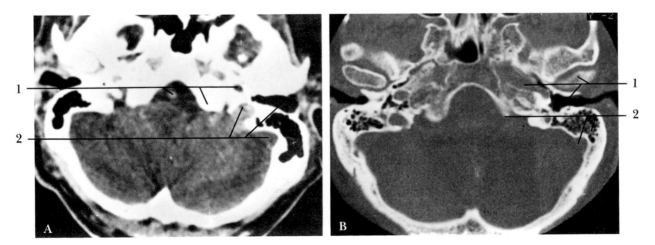

FIG. 10.8. Normal CT images at approximately the same level through the lower posterior fossa. **A.** Normal CT image. *1,* Carotid canal, jugular tubercle, large vertebral artery; *2,* sigmoid sinus, external auditory meatus, jugular foramen. **B.** Bone window image. *1,* Carotid canal, mandible, external auditory meatus; *2,* jugular tubercle, sigmoid sinus, mastoid air cells.

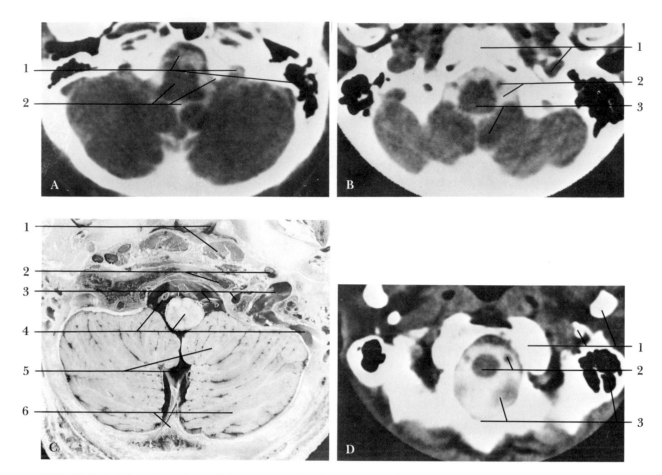

FIG. 10.9. Axial sections through lower posterior fossa. **A.** CT cisternogram. *1*, Jugular fossa, mastoid air cells, medullary cistern with tortuous vessels; *2*, fourth ventricle in front of tonsils, jugular tubercle, medulla. **B.** CT cisternogram. *1*, Clivus, jugular foramen; *2*, vertebral artery, medullary cistern with rootlets of vagus; *3*, closed medulla, tonsil, mastoid air cells. **C.** Anatomic section. *1*, Nasopharynx, longus colli muscle; *2*, internal carotid artery, clivus; *3*, jugular foramen, hypoglossal canal, hypoglossal rootlets; *4*, sigmoid sinus, medulla, right vertebral artery; *5*, cisterna magna, tonsil; *6*, cerebellar hemisphere, internal occipital protuberance. **D.** CT cisternogram. *1*, Condyle, styloid process, mandible; *2*, closed medulla, left vertebral artery; *3*, posterior rim of foramen magnum, tonsil (averaged-in), mastoid air cells.

tions (Fig. 10.13). The *vertebral arteries* are seen far lateral in the *transverse foramina;* the *cord* at the level of C1 and C2 is slightly smaller in diameter than in lower cervical sections.

Magnetic resonance images just below the foramen magnum clearly demonstrate large vessels, muscles, fat, and fascial compartments (Fig. 10.14); however, the details of the spinal cord with its rootlets are less well seen. The absence of artifacts is again noted. The advantage of MR in the craniovertebral junction lies not only in the ability to show anatomic relationships, but also in the demonstration of flow in the major vessels; when certain set-

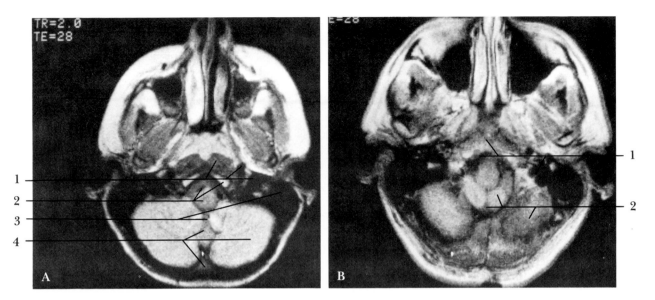

FIG. 10.10. MR images (spin echo) through lower posterior fossa (two different persons). **A.** *1*, Jugular vein, internal carotid artery, longus colli muscle; *2*, closed medulla, occipital condyle, right vertebral artery; *3*, mastoid process, median aperture; *4*, cerebellar hemisphere, lower vermis between tonsils, internal occipital protuberance. **B.** *1*, Vertebral artery in medullary cistern, clivus, jugular bulb; *2*, cisterna magna, tonsil, cerebellar hemisphere.

tings are used, the fast-flowing blood in the vessel appears black (no signal), vascular occlusions appear gray (intermediate signal), and turbulence or slow flow in a vessel appears whitish (strong signal). Note in Figure 10.14 the presence of a retention cyst in the right maxillary sinus.

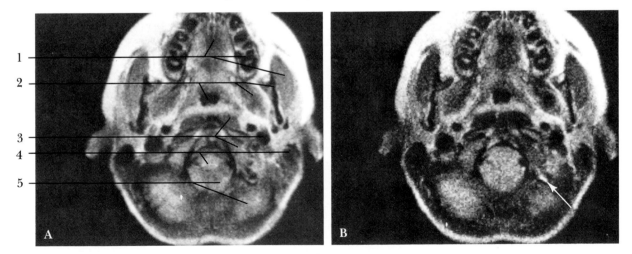

FIG. 10.11. Normal MR (spin echo) images through the foramen magnum obtained with different spin echo parameters. **A.** First echo. *1*, Maxilla with teeth, masseter muscle, hard palate; *2*, mandible, pterygoid muscles, nasopharynx; *3*, jugular foramen, occipital condyle, longus colli muscle; *4*, mastoid process, medulla; *5*, tonsil, cerebellar hemisphere. **B.** Second echo. The vessels are seen more clearly due to the high-signal CSF (long T2); a slow-flowing vein *(arrow)* has a high-signal intensity.

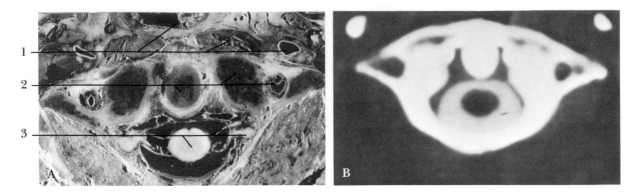

FIG. 10.12. Images through the lateral masses of C1. **A.** Anatomic section. *1*, Internal carotid artery, longus colli muscle, nasopharynx; *2*, vertebral artery, lateral mass of C1, dens; *3*, dorsal root ganglion of C2, motor root, spinal cord. **B.** Corresponding CT cisternogram.

Altered Anatomy Pathologic processes are classified, here, as elsewhere in the lower regions of the spine, as extradural, intradural, extramedullary, and intramedullary (which of course is intradural). These distinctions are of considerable importance for the strategies of treatment and for prognosis. In the upper cervical region, where the subarachnoid space is wide, the distinction is sometimes difficult to make on CT images, despite cisternography; an example of an intradural, extramedullary mass is shown in Figure 10.15 (compare with Fig. 10.6B). Pre-operatively, the mass was thought to be extradural in nature.

The advantage of CT in the diagnosis and analysis of traumatic conditions of the upper spine is illustrated in Figure 10.16: the patient was admitted to the emergency room with a twisted

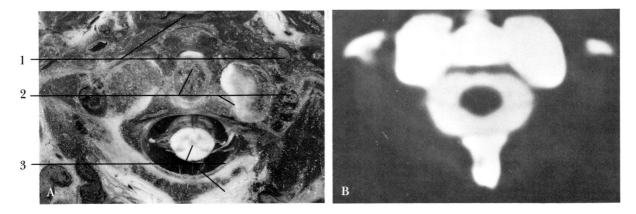

FIG. 10.13. Axial images at the level of the atlanto-occipital joint. **A.** Anatomic section. *1*, Carotid artery, nasopharynx; *2*, vertebral artery, atlanto-axial joint, dens; *3*, dura, posterior element of C2, cord. **B.** Corresponding CT image.

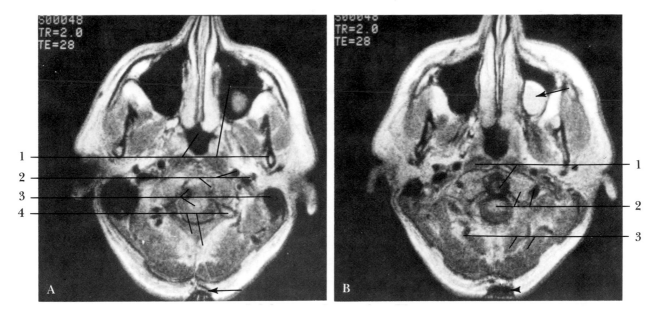

FIG. 10.14. MR images (spin echo) just below foramen magnum. **A.** *1*, Mandible, maxillary air sinus, nasopharynx; *2*, jugular vein, internal carotid artery, condyle; *3*, mastoid process, cord, right vertebral artery; *4*, veins, suboccipital fat, posterior arch of C1. **B.** Slightly lower. *1*, Longus colli muscle, odontoid process, branch of external carotid artery; *2*, cord, lateral mass of C1, vertebral artery; *3*, deep cervical vein, suboccipital muscles. A retention cyst is present within the maxillary air sinus *(arrow)*. There is a "fold-over" artifact *(arrowhead)* in both images because the nose is too long for the image size.

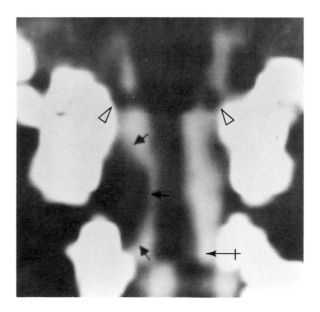

FIG. 10.15. Coronal reformation of a series of axial CT cisternograms of the craniovertebral junction region. A mass *(arrows)* is seen lateral to the cord; the vertebral arteries *(arrowheads)* lie along the medulla. Movement off-set *(crossed arrow)* in lower part of image.

neck and quadriparesis, which was shown to be caused by rotatory C1/C2 subluxation that was not clearly defined on plain films.

Clinical Cases
Case 18

A 2-year-old, white, male child was referred because of renal failure, hypertension, and seizures. A sibling with similar S/S had died a year earlier. Pregnancy and birth were uncomplicated. Normal development had occurred until 6 months ago, when growth slowed and head size seemed abnormally large. When the child was 10 months old, a ventriculogram and arteriogram were done. (Radiology report was unobtainable.) He walked at 20 months, talked at 22 months.

Three months PTA Pt developed hypertension (190/100); 2 months PTA he developed HA, followed by acute right hemiplegia, and a brief seizure. What is your DDX at this time?

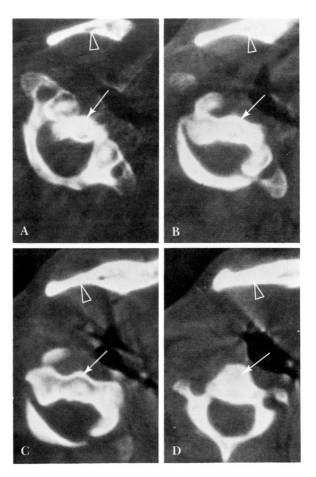

FIG. 10.16. Serial CT images to show traumatic, rotatory subluxation of C2 *(arrows)* in relation to C1 and the left mandible *(arrowheads)*. (Courtesy of Dr. M. Brant-Zawadski)

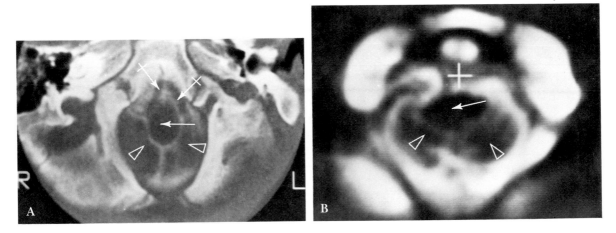

FIG. 10.17. Axial CT cisternograms at the craniovertebral junction. **A.** Thick section of the level of the foramen magnum. The tonsils *(arrowheads)*, medulla *(arrow)*, and vertebral arteries *(crossed arrows)* are visible. **B.** Level of the occipital condyles. The tonsils *(arrowheads)* are seen behind the enlarged cord diameter *(arrow)*.

> GPE: Hgt, 80 cm; Wgt, 10.9 kg; head circumference, 52 cm. BP, 155/95; liver, spleen palpable. An intern had noted a soft swelling at the nape of the neck, not confirmed on later exams.

> NEX: Irritable, understood commands, made appropriate responses, spoke simple phrases. No papilledema; PERRL, EOMs intact.

> *Motor system:* grossly symm., DTRs 2 +.

> *Sensory system:* Nl.

> A CT study was performed (Fig. 10.17). What are your findings? DX?

> (Discussion of Case 18 and additional illustrations on p. 214.)

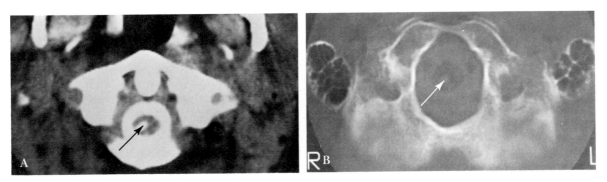

FIG. 10.18. CT cisternograms at the level of the craniovertebral junction. **A.** Soft tissue settings. The high density within the cord *(arrow)* is at the level of C1. **B.** Bone window image at the level of the foramen magnum. Note the high density within the cord *(arrow)*.

CASE 19 A 24-year-old female camp counselor was admitted to the hospital with complaints of progressive weakness in the legs. Her skin seemed wet, although she did not run a temperature. Her speech appeared thick.

GPX: Hyperhydrosis of the entire body below the neck. BP: some degree of postural hypotension.

NEX: MS wnl.

CNN: Weakness of the tongue in all directions.

Motor system: increased spasticity and weakness of the LEs, less severe in the UEs.

Sensory system: loss of sense of pain and temperature mostly over the entire lower body; position and vibratory sense intact.

Spine films were normal except for a minimal subluxation at the level of C5. What additional neurodiagnostic procedures would be useful? A CT scan with intrathecal contrast was done, and repeated 6 hours later (Fig. 10.18). What are your findings? What is your DDX?
(Discussion of Case 19 on p. 215.)

Questions 10a. Which structures pass through the jugular foramen?

10b. What is the procedure of choice (using CT) to demonstrate the precise diameter of the cord?

10c. Why is a CT cisternogram (or an MR study if possible) useful in determining the site of lesions in the region of the craniovertebral junction?

10d. What is the potential location of an intradural, extramedullary mass? Is it in the subdural space? In the subarachnoid space? In either? In both?

10e. Which ligament prevents (sub)luxation of the odontoid process of the axis (C2) away from the anterior arch of the atlas (C1)?

10f. What is the main movement possible in the atlanto-axial articulation? Which is the principal movement in the atlanto-occipital joint?

11. Cervical and Thoracic Spine

Cervical Spine

The five lower cervical vertebrae, together with the atlas (C1) and axis (C2) form a portion of the spinal column that is characterized by high mobility, by its relationship with the vertebral arteries, and by the emergence of most of the brachial plexus.

NORMAL VERTEBRAL MORPHOLOGY

Each lower cervical vertebra has a wide *vertebral canal* that is roughly triangular in shape (Fig. 11.1). The *transverse processes* are small; they contain anteriorly *costal elements,* and a *foramen transversarium* for the vertebral artery and veins on each side. These transverse foramina may be equal or different in size; sometimes a bony septum is present within a foramen, separating the artery from the veins. The transverse foramina may be absent altogether, a condition that is rare in C2 to C6, but not infrequent in C7. The transverse process is usually larger in C7 than in higher vertebrae because the costal elements are more developed; these elements may occasionally form a "cervical rib" on one or both sides. The *spinous processes* of the lower cervical vertebrae tend to be bifid (Fig. 11.5A), except in C7; this lowermost cervical vertebra has a long and well-developed spinous process ("vertebra prominens") that normally is easily palpable (Fig. 11.1; see also Figs. 11.4A and 11.5A). Sometimes the spinous process of T1 is even more prominent, however.

The *bodies* of the lower five cervical vertebrae are relatively small, convex anteriorly and concave posteriorly, with two lateral ridges on the upper surfaces, the *uncinate processes* (Figs. 11.1 and 11.2). There is a corresponding rounding on each side of the lower surfaces of C3 to C6. The *intervertebral discs* are therefore relatively small and squared-off (Fig. 11.2). The result of this arrangement of the stack of cervical bodies with their uncinate processes is that lateral movement is restricted, but flexion or

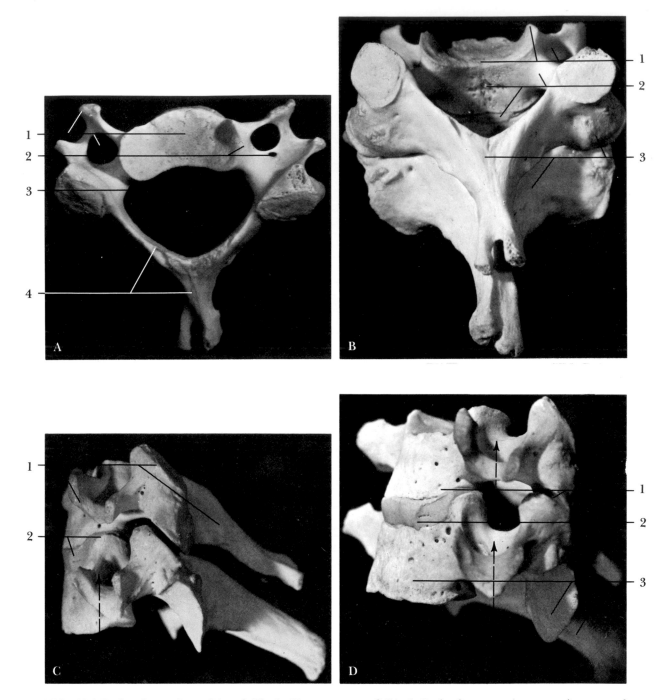

FIG. 11.1 Isolated vertebrae C4 and C5. **A.** Upper aspect of C4. *1*, Body, foramen transversarium, costal elements; *2*, uncinate process, accessory foramen transversarium; *3*, lateral recess, superior articular facet; *4*, spinous process, laminae. **B.** C4 and C5 viewed obliquely from behind and above. *1*, Endplate of body, uncinate process, foramen transversarium; *2*, opening for basivertebral vein, intervertebral disc, pedicle; *3*, spinous process, lamina of C5, inferior articular process of C4. **C.** Lateral view. *1*, Superior articular facet, spinous process, costal elements of C4; *2*, disc, uncinate process; *arrow* through foramen transversarium of C5. **D.** Oblique anterior view. *1*, Uncinate process, facet joint; *2*, disc, intervertebral foramen; *3*, body, inferior articular process, spinous process of C5 (*arrows* pass through foramina transversaria).

extension is quite easy. The articular processes lie lateral to the *laminae,* and behind the *pedicles;* the *articular facets* (superior and inferior) slope slightly downward (Figs. 11.1B and C). This oblique coronal orientation of the *facet joint* is different from that in the thoracic and lumbar spine; the movements of flexion and extension are easy in the C-spine.

The relationships of the vertebra, its processes, and the *intervertebral disc* to the *dural (thecal) sac,* the *intervertebral foramen,* and the *nerve roots* are shown in Figure 11.2. The plane of section is slightly up anteriorly; hence the bony endplate of the next higher vertebra appears to lie in front of the disc. It should be noted that the intervertebral foramina are situated between the pedicles of the vertebrae above and below, and between the uncinate processes medially and the articulations laterally. Since the cervical spinal nerves pass through these intervertebral foramina, hypertrophy of the joint facets, spondylosis, osteophytes, or disc herniation may diminish the size of a foramen and encroach on the spinal nerve and its dorsal root ganglion.

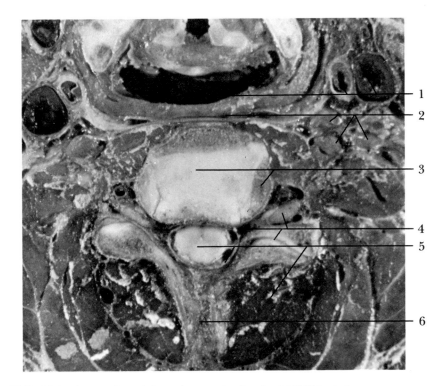

FIG. 11.2. Anatomic axial section at the level of C5/C6. *1,* Larynx, common carotid, internal jugular vein; *2,* esophagus (collapsed), brachial plexus; *3,* disc, uncinate process; *4,* vein, facet joint, dorsal root ganglion; *5,* cord, dura, paraspinous muscles; *6,* spinous process.

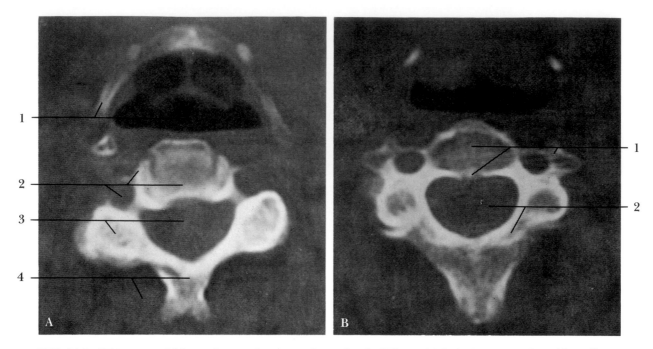

FIG. 11.3. CT images of thin sections at the approximate level of Figure 11.2. **A.** *1*, Larynx, thyroid cartilage; *2*, endplate of C6, uncinate process, foramen transversarium; *3*, vertebral canal, articular pillar; *4*, spinous process, paraspinous muscles. **B.** Slightly higher than Figure 11.3a. *1*, Body of C5, basivertebral vein, costal elements; *2*, vertebral canal, lamina.

Two CT images, corresponding to Figure 11.2, with a wide window setting not only demonstrate the shape of the vertebral body with its uncinate processes quite well, but also the triangular or heart-shaped, wide vertebral canal at the midcervical level (Fig. 11.3). Such images depict the skeletal details well: the technique is quite useful in evaluating trauma to the spine. However, visualization of the intradural spaces and structures (cord, nerve roots) requires the injection of a contrast solution, usually administered by lumbar puncture, occasionally by a puncture at the C1-C2 level.

NEURAL
ELEMENTS

Figure 11.4 contains a series of thin sections with intrathecal contrast, demonstrating the normal bony and soft-tissue elements in and around the cervical vertebral canal. Note the forward convergence of the *nerve roots* through the lateral recesses into the intervertebral foramina; the anterior median fissure of the *cord* is visible. There is an anterior *epidural space,* in which the anterior *veins* course, as well as the posterior longitudinal ligament (normally not identifiable). At the posterior midbody level, one or two *basivertebral veins* connect the venous channels within the body with the anterior epidural veins, which communicate with systemic veins outside the vertebrae. This arrangement, present in the cervical region save in C1, occurs throughout the vertebral column. The posterior epidural space contains veins, the ligamenta flava, and little or no fat. If the anterior epidural veins

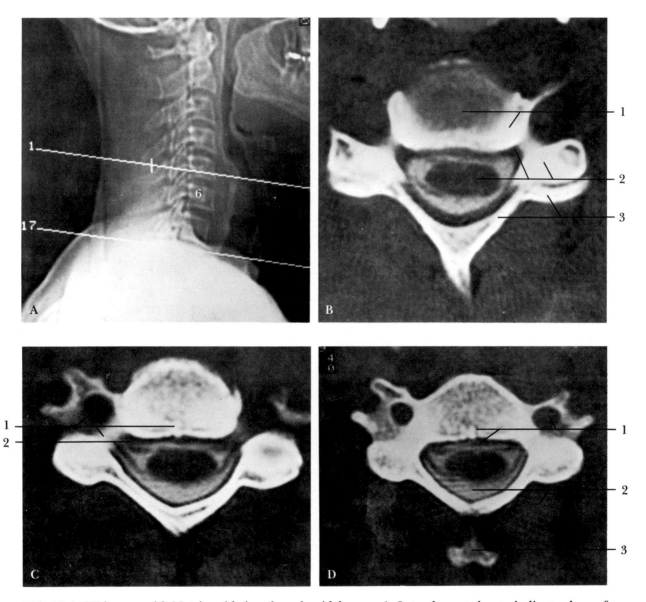

FIG. 11.4. CT images with Metrizamide in subarachnoidal space. **A.** Lateral scout view to indicate plane of thin sections. **B.** Level of the C5/C6 disc. *1*, Disc, uncinate process; *2*, cord, lateral recess, superior articular process of C5; *3*, lamina, inferior articular process of C5. **C.** Across the upper endplate of C6. *1*, Body, intervertebral foramen above pedicle, foramen for vertebral artery; *2*, anterior and posterior roots. **D.** Level of the middle of C6. *1*, Basivertebral vein, extradural space, foramen transversarium; *2*, contrast in subarachnoid space, paraspinous muscles; *3*, spinous process of C5. (Courtesy of Dr. D. LaMasters)

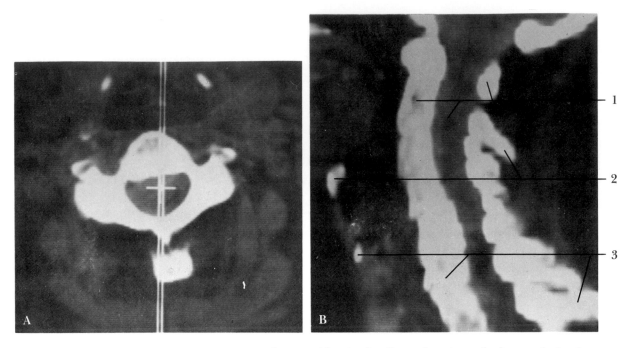

FIG. 11.5. Approximate midsagittal reformation through the cervical spine. **A.** Plane of CT reformation. **B.** *1*, Body of C2, vertebral canal, posterior arch of C1; *2*, hyoid, spinous process of C2; *3*, calcified thyroid cartilage, body of C6, spinous process of C7.

are engorged, the resulting bulge into the dura may faintly resemble a central *herniation* of the *nucleus pulposus*. The normally occurring venous channels within the vertebral body, converging into the basivertebral vein, have been mistaken for fractures on thin-section CT images.

A sagittal CT reformation can be very useful to define the limits and shape of the vertebral canal in cases of suspected disc herniations, or to determine if free disc fragments are present. A reformation may demonstrate traumatic dislocations more clearly. When tumors are suspected, either within the spinal canal or elsewhere in the vertebral region, CT reformations can be of great value to the neurosurgeon by showing the location, size, and shape of the mass. Figure 11.5 shows such a reformation, in a slightly parasagittal plane in a normal person.

One of the great advantages of MR over CT is that an image can be obtained *directly,* in almost any desired plane (Fig. 11.6). The soft tissues around the vertebral column are demonstrated with the same detail, which may be an added advantage in the event that large lesions extend beyond the spine. Computed tomography images in the lower neck region are often degraded by the presence of the shoulders unless special precautions are taken. However, the quality of bone detail in CT images is usually better than in MR images.

Anatomic axial or CT images at the level of the larynx demonstrate the cervical vertebrae as well as the adjacent soft tissues (Fig. 11.7). Even when bone window settings are used the anatomic and fascial relationships and planes in the neck are visible (Fig. 11.7C).

Thoracic Spine

NORMAL VERTEBRAL MORPHOLOGY

The thoracic vertebrae are characterized by a *round vertebral canal,* an anteriorly round, posteriorly concave *body,* a well-developed pair of transverse processes with articular facets for the ribs, and long, slender, down-sloping *spinous processes* that overlie each other like roof shingles (Fig. 11.8). The *articular facets* lie in an approximately true coronal plane. Anteroflexion and lateral bending movements are easier performed than dorsiflexion, be-

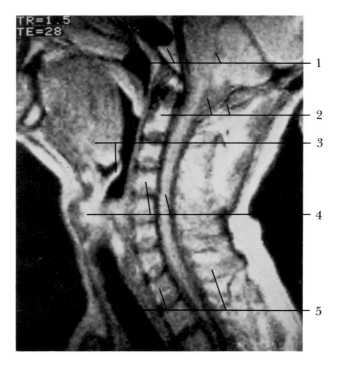

FIG. 11.6. Direct midsagittal MR (spin echo) image through the craniovertebral junction and neck. *1,* Nasopharynx, clivus, fourth ventricle; *2,* C2, cisterna magna, occiput; *3,* tongue, epiglottis, oropharynx; *4,* larynx, C4 vertebra, cord; *5,* trachea, T1 body, C7 spinous process. The cord margins are clearly seen without intrathecal contrast (first echo image).

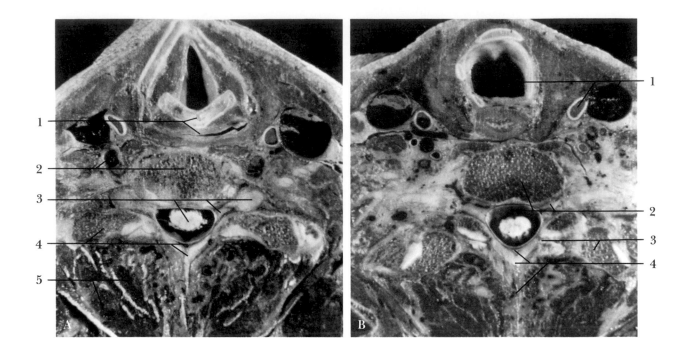

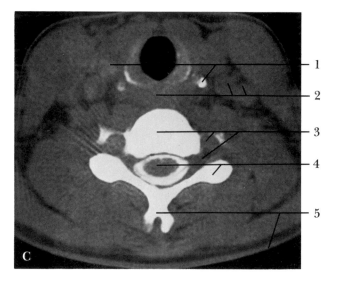

FIG. 11.7. Axial sections through the lower C-spine. **A.** Anatomic section. *1*, Arytenoid cartilage, esophagus, jugular vein; *2*, body of C6, vertebral artery; *3*, cord, nerve roots, dorsal root ganglion; *4*, epidural space, ligamentum flavum, transverse process; *5*, paraspinous musculature. **B.** Anatomic section. *1*, Trachea, common carotid, jugular vein; *2*, subarachnoid space, body of C7, intervertebral foramen; *3*, facet joint, transverse process; *4*, epidural fat, ligamentum flavum, interspinous ligament. **C.** CT image. *1*, Calcification in thyroid gland, trachea, calcified thyroid cartilage; *2*, esophagus, carotid, jugular vein; *3*, body of C6, foramen transversarium, intervertebral foramen; *4*, cord within intrathecal contrast column, articular pillar; *5*, spinous process, skin.

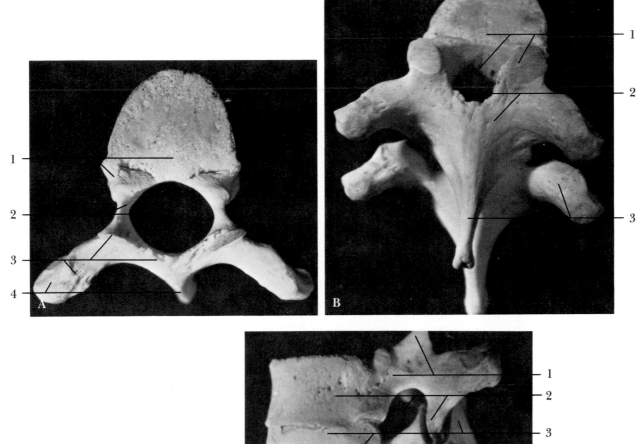

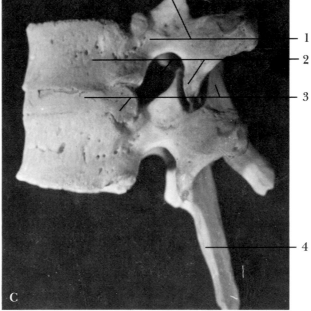

FIG. 11.8. Vertebrae T4 and T5. **A.** Superior view of T4. *1*, Upper endplate, costovertebral joint facet; *2*, vertebral canal, pedicle; *3*, lamina, superior articular facet, transverse process; *4*, spinous process, costotransversal joint facet. **B.** Superior oblique view. *1*, Body of T4, basivertebral vein opening, superior articular facet; *2*, vertebral canal, lamina, costotransversal joint facet; *3*, spinous process of T4, transverse process of T5. **C.** Lateral view. *1*, Pedicle, superior articular facet; *2*, body of T4, intervertebral foramen, inferior articular process; *3*, disc, costovertebral joint facet (artificially filled), spinous process of T4; *4*, spinous process of T5.

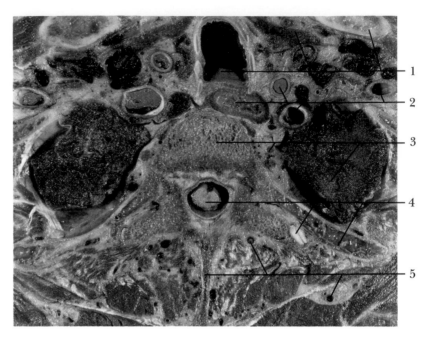

FIG. 11.9. Anatomic axial section at the level of the lung apices. *1*, Trachea, thyroid gland, clavicle; *2*, esophagus, common carotid, subclavian artery (twice); *3*, body of T2, spinal nerve, lung; *4*, cord, costotransverse joint, rib; *5*, spinous process, deep thoracic veins.

cause of the shape of the facet joints. The *pedicles* are larger than in the cervical spine; the *intervertebral foramen* is contained anteriorly by the body and disc, superiorly and inferiorly by the pedicles of the adjacent vertebrae, and posteriorly by the facet joint.

Epidural fat is present posteriorly within the vertebral canal of the thoracic spine but is hardly present in the cervical spine. An *epidural venous plexus* is present at all levels, in communication with one or two *basivertebral* veins that emerge from the middle of the posterior aspect of the vertebral bodies similar to the distribution in the cervical spine (Figs. 11.9, 11.10, and 11.11). The anterior epidural venous plexus is continuous with the cervical plexus and the basilar plexus of the posterior fossa, as well as with the lumbar epidural plexus. The thoracic epidural plexus communicates with the radicular veins (Fig. 11.11).

DIAMETER OF THE SPINAL CORD

The spinal cord is oval in diameter and widens in the region between the fifth cervical and first thoracic segments, where the many thick, down-sloping rootlets ultimately form the brachial plexus (see Figs. 11.3, 11.4, and 11.7). In the thoracic region, the cord is round and smaller in diameter than in the C-spine (Figs.

11.8A and 11.11). The normal anteroposterior diameter does not vary much between C1 and C7 (6 to 7 mm); the lateral diameter, however, increases from 7 mm at C1 to 12 mm at C7. The thoracic cord is round with a 6-mm diameter. It is important to realize that the cervical enlargement within the vertebral canal begins about 15-mm higher than the position of the (C5/C6) intervertebral foramen. This normal increase in diameter should be distinguished from an intramedullary (intradural) mass leading to enlargement of the cord at an abnormal level.

Altered Anatomy

Figure 11.12A shows an abnormal anatomic relationship between the body of a vertebra and the vertebral canal; the foramina transversaria appear too wide and are no longer surrounded

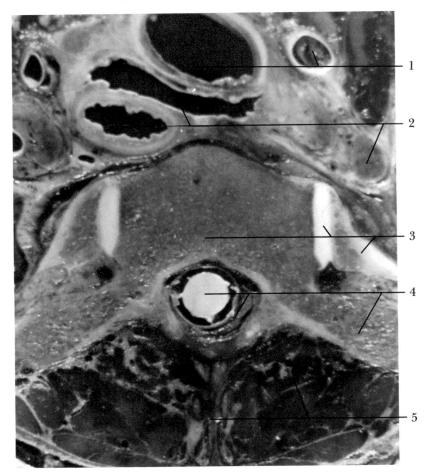

FIG. 11.10. Anatomic axial section through upper T-spine. *1*, Trachea, common carotid; *2*, esophagus, artifact, hilar lymph node; *3*, body of T3, costovertebral joint, rib head; *4*, cord, extradural space, transverse process; *5*, interspinous ligament, paraspinous muscles.

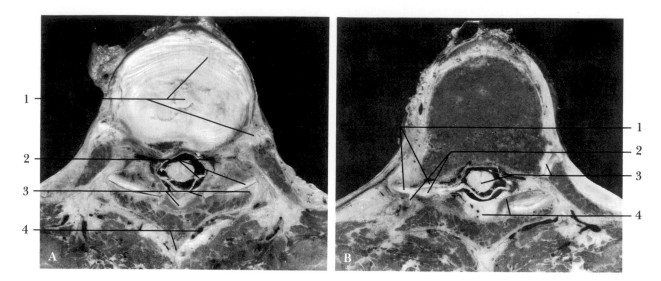

FIG. 11.11. Axial sections through middle T-spine preparations. **A.** *1*, Nucleus pulposus, annulus fibrosus, costovertebral joint; *2*, anterior extradural vein, facet joint, dura; *3*, articular process, ligamentum flavum, epidural fat; *4*, base of spinous process, deep veins. **B.** *1*, Ventral root, ventral ramus; *2*, dorsal root ganglion, dorsal ramus; *3*, cord, epidural vein, costovertebral joint; *4*, epidural fat, ligamentum flavum blending with joint capsule.

by bone. The patient was quadriparetic after a severe accident. The explanation of the abnormal anatomy is given in a lateral view (a plain film here, rather than a CT reformation). The diagnosis was C6-C7 subluxation causing compression of the spinal cord and roots.

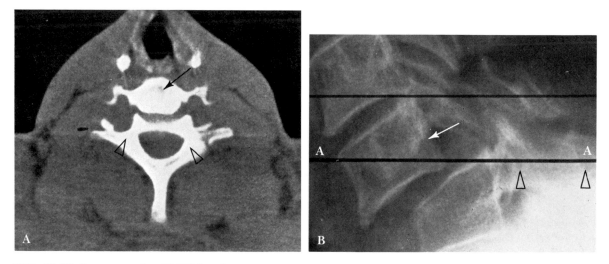

FIG. 11.12. Images at the C6/C7 level. **A.** Axial CT scan. C6 body *(arrow)* lies anterior to elements of C7 *(arrowheads)*. **B.** Lateral spine film. C6 body *(arrow)* has been displaced anteriorly, so that elements of C7 lie behind in a plane A-A (corresponding to Figure 11.12A). (Courtesy of Dr. M. Brant-Zawadski)

Figure 11.13 shows a condition often seen in elderly patients, less severe than the previous case, yet producing neurologic deficits. There is considerable spondylosis with formation of osteophytes narrowing the intervertebral foramina. In addition, there is calcification of the posterior longitudinal ligament (clearly demonstrable on midsagittal reformations). Such spinal stenosis with narrow foramina may cause severe pain; however, the neurosurgeon can give considerable relief by enlarging the intervertebral foramina (often necessary at several levels).

A so-called "seatbelt" fracture is seen in Figure 11.14. The upper anterior margin of T12 is cracked off with free bone fragments present; the body of T12 has become displaced posteriorly. The parallel high densities, high in the vertebral canal, represent a contrast column blocked at T12. The subluxation and fractures can best be demonstrated on a sagittal reformation as seen in Figure 11.14. This type of trauma may occur in high-speed collisions when a shoulder restraint is not available or is not used. The spinal cord is compressed, resulting in paraplegia; however, without *any* belt, the patient most likely would have been even more seriously injured, or killed.

A sagittal MR image can demonstrate the extent of intraspinal lesions directly (Fig. 11.15). A mass (metastasis of renal cell

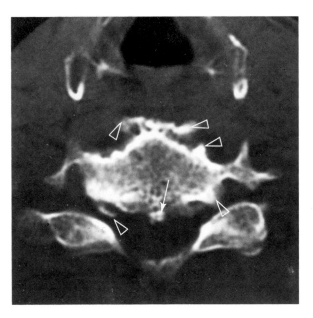

FIG. 11.13. CT image at the level of C5. Spondylotic changes *(arrowheads)*, calcified posterior longitudinal ligament *(arrow)*, resulting in canal stenosis and narrowing of the intervertebral foramina.

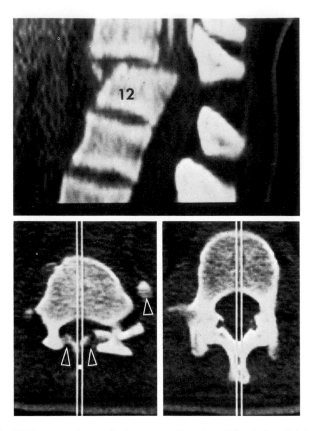

FIG. 11.14. CT images through the lower T-spine. The left axial image shows fractures *(arrowheads)*; the right axial image appears normal. There is a total block at T11/T12 of the intrathecal contrast column, and the cord is compressed. (Federle, M.P., and Brant-Zawadski, M. (eds.): Computed Tomography in the Evaluation of Trauma. Baltimore, Williams & Wilkins, 1982.)

carcinoma) on T11 is seen in relation to the surrounding structures and spaces. The cord is compressed. Note the aorta anterior to the vertebral column.

Clinical Cases

CASE 20

A 30-year-old man visited his doctor with a complaint of loss of sensation in three fingers of each hand. Five years previously the patient had become aware of some stiffness in his neck over the L posterior aspect. He also noticed a "snapping feeling" on turning to the extreme left or right. This condition remained static with perhaps some lessening of the neck pain until 4 months PTA. At that time, the patient noted that neck extension would produce numbness or tingling in the two ulnar fingers of both hands and possibly the toes of both feet. He had also noted slight weakness of all extremities, with a loss of coordination when writing (the weakness had increased in recent months). He felt a "shooting" pain in his L arm when sneezing or coughing.

NEX: MS and CNN: Intact.

Motor system: Weakness of the L triceps and of the extensors of the L wrist; some weakness of abduction of the fingers. Weakness in dorsiflexion of the toes; gait slightly spastic and ataxic with a tendency to circumduct the L leg.

DTRs: L biceps and radial decreased; triceps increased. Quadriceps and Achilles tendon increased L more than R, with some ankle clonus bilaterally. Extensor plantar responses bilaterally.

Sensory system: Vibration and position sense decreased, absent in the fifth, fourth, and middle fingers. Pain sense slightly decreased on the L side.

What is your preliminary DDX? What neurodiagnostic procedure would you have done?

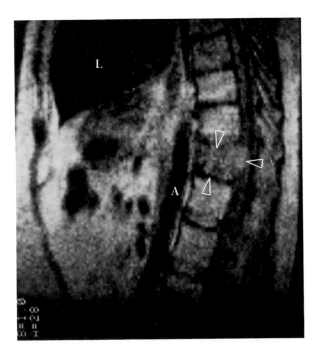

FIG. 11.15. Direct mid-sagittal MR image (spin echo). The enlarged vertebral body of T11 *(arrowheads)* forms an anterior extradural mass (renal cell carcinoma metastasis). There is gas in the large and small bowels. *A* = aorta; *L* = liver.

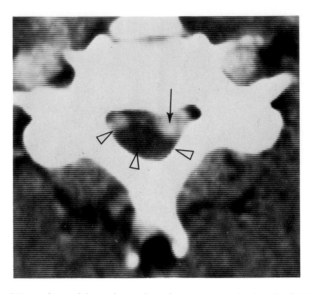

FIG. 11.16. CT section without intrathecal contrast at the level of C6. The dural sac *(arrowheads)* is compressed by a left centrolateral disc *(arrow)*.

Plain spine films wnl. CT with intrathecal contrast was done, with a representative section at C5/C6 in Figure 11.16. Now what is your DX?

(Discussion of Case 20 and additional illustrations on p. 216.)

CASE 21   A 33-year-old man was referred to a neurologist because of complaints of gradually increasing weakness and decrease in pain sensation in the legs, and weakness in his R triceps.

NEX: Well-developed man with some atrophy in the R triceps compared to L; forearm kept semiflexed.

Motor system: Wrist-drop, loss of strength in triceps; L and R leg muscles weak, both flexors and extensors (more so on the L).

Sensory system: Loss of pain and temperature sensation on the R side of the body up to mamillary level, L side wnl. Some loss of position sense in the R LE.

A plain spine film was entirely normal. A CT study with intrathecal contrast was performed (Fig. 11.17). What are your findings? What is your DDX?

(Discussion of Case 21 and additional illustrations on p. 216.)

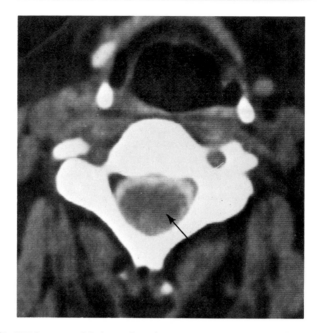

FIG. 11.17. CT image with intrathecal contrast at the level of C5; the cord is enlarged *(arrow)*.

Questions   11a. What is the difference in articular facet orientation between the cervical and thoracic spine?

11b. What would be the functional importance of the uncinate processes in the cervical spine?

11c. How can the intradural contents be visualized best, using CT?

11d. At which spinal cord level is the cord largest in diameter? At which cord level is the vertebral canal widest?

11e. Lateral cervical spondylosis may cause pain or weakness, or both, when the ipsilateral arm is elevated; what is a possible explanation for this?

11f. Which spinal nerve emerges through the C5/C6 intervertebral foramen? Which spinal nerve emerges through the T5/T6 intervertebral foramen?

12. Lumbosacral Spine

The availability of high-resolution CT with reformations has led, in recent years, to a general acceptance of CT for diagnostic studies of the lumbosacral region. Myelography readily provides spatial and longitudinal information on the condition of intrathecal contents (cord, meninges, nerve roots); however, this procedure gives only indirect clues concerning the shape and size of normal structures or pathologic processes that are immediately adjacent to and outside the dura. More remote areas cannot be evaluated with myelographic methods.

Consecutive, high resolution, thin transaxial CT scans now provide the most accurate, easiest, and fastest information, not only of the dura and contents, but also of the condition of the bony structures, joints, ligaments, spinal nerves, etc. The combination of CT with preceding injection of water-soluble contrast into the subarachnoid space is the most complete and informative procedure to date for the examination of the lumbosacral region. An understanding of the anatomic relationships of this region is essential. Magnetic resonance images in this region are (so far) limited in resolution, although quite helpful in some cases.

Normal Anatomy

LUMBAR VERTEBRAL MORPHOLOGY

The five lumbar vertebrae are the largest elements of the spinal column; the sacrum represents five fused vertebrae, in which thin intervertebral discs are normally present. Occasionally, the fifth lumbar vertebra has become fused with the sacrum on one or both sides ("sacralization of L5"). The large *bodies* of L1 through L5 are stout, oval structures with normally a slightly concave posterior surface, except L5 (Figs. 12.1 and 12.2). The lumbar *intervertebral* discs have a similar shape: they are thinner pos-

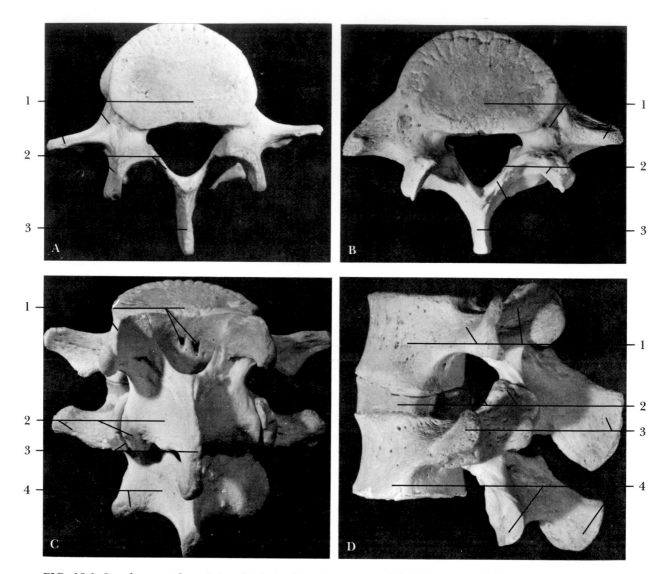

FIG. 12.1. Lumbar vertebrae L4 and L5. **A.** Superior aspect of L4. *1,* upper endplate, pedicle, transverse process; *2,* vertebral canal, lamina, superior articular facet; *3,* spinous process. **B.** Superior aspect of L5. *1,* Upper endplate, pedicle, transverse process; *2,* vertebral canal, artifact, superior articular facet; *3,* spinous process, lamina. **C.** View from behind and above. *1,* Upper endplate, openings for basivertebral veins, superior articular process; *2,* lamina, inferior articular process of L4, transverse process of L5; *3,* spinous process of L4, facet joint; *4,* lamina, inferior articular process of L5. **D.** Lateral view. *1,* body, pedicle, superior articular process of L4; *2,* disc, intervertebral foramen, superior articular process of L5; *3,* transverse process, spinous process of L4; *4,* body of L5, inferior articular facet, spinous process.

teriorly than anteriorly, a feature that contributes to the physiologic lumbar lordosis.

The *transverse processes* are relatively thin; the *spinous processes,* however, are large quadrangular bony plates that slope slightly downwards (Fig. 12.1D). An articular pillar contains the

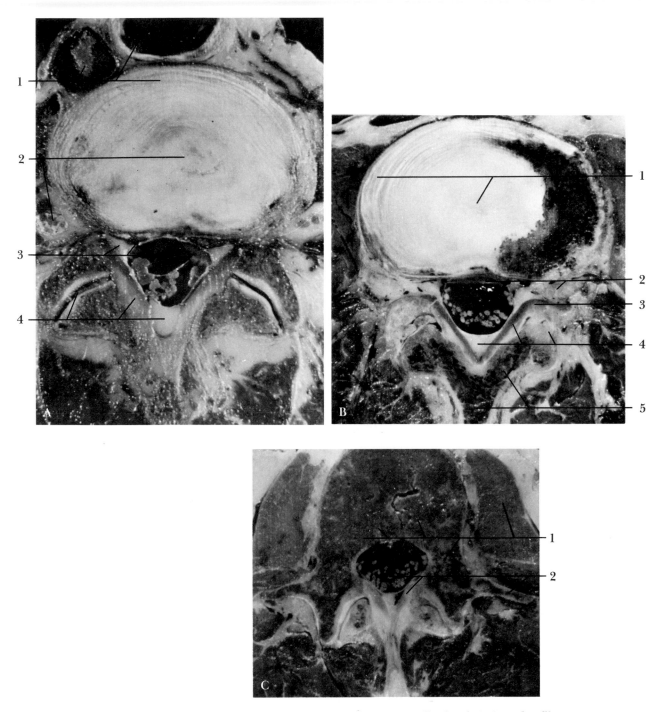

FIG. 12.2 Anatomic axial sections through lumbar vertebrae. **A.** L3/L4 disc level. *1*, Annulus fibrosus, aorta, inferior vena cava; *2*, nucleus pulposus, spinal nerve branches; *3*, dural sac, epidural vein, lateral recess with fat; *4*, epidural fat, ligamentum flavum, facet joint. **B.** Slightly oblique section through L4 endplate and L4/L5 disc. *1*, Annulus fibrosus, nucleus pulposus, endplate; *2*, epidural vein, cauda equina, dorsal root ganglion; *3*, ligamentum flavum blending with facet joint capsule; *4*, epidural fat, ligamentum flavum, superior articular process; *5*, spinous process, lamina. **C.** Body of L4 level. *1*, Body, pedicle, psoas; *2*, cauda equina, ligamentum flavum, transverse process.

lumbar *articulations* formed by superior and inferior processes, with respectively concave and convex *articular facets;* the facet *joints* are oriented in an oblique plane halfway between the coronal and parasagittal planes (Fig. 12.1C and 12.2). The lumbar *laminae* are short and wide, unlike the thoracic laminae (compare Fig. 11.8 with 12.1). The *pedicles* form stout bridges between the upper half of the vertebral bodies and the posterior elements. Note that the *intervertebral foramen* is confined by the adjacent pedicles above and below; by the body and intervertebral disc anteriorly, and by the articular pillar posteriorly (Fig. 12.1D). One or more foramina may be reduced in size (thereby compromising the spinal nerve and dorsal root ganglion) by a number of pathologic conditions: encroachment of a herniated ("slipped") disc; hyperostosis of the articular processes; traumatic displacement of bone fragments; osteophytes, which occur often in elderly people; and congenital narrowing of the foramina.

NEURAL
ELEMENTS

The *nerve root pairs* (ventral and dorsal root on each side) leave the *cauda equina* by moving into the lateral recesses, then exiting through the intervertebral foramen just below the pedicles of the vertebra with the same number (Fig. 12.1D and 12.2): L1 nerves are found in the L1/L2 intervertebral spaces, L2 nerves in the L2/L3 spaces, and so on.

The soft tissues related to the lumbar vertebrae are illustrated in Figure 12.2: large vessels anteriorly, psoas muscles anterolaterally, and paraspinous musculature posterolaterally. Within the vertebral canal the dural sac with its nerve roots is normally imbedded in extradural fat, especially posteriorly and in the lateral recesses. As at other spinal levels, the ligamentum flavum is present between the laminae of adjacent vertebrae; it blends with the joint capsules anteriorly (Fig. 12.2). The relationships of the nerve roots and spinal nerves are illustrated in Figure 12.3.

A series of thin, normal CT scans illustrates the bony elements, spaces, intradural nerves, and filum terminale (internum) quite well, especially after intrathecal contrast injection, using a bone window setting (Fig. 12.4). These normal contours and relationships of disc, dura, and intervertebral space should be scrutinized carefully; flattening or bulging of the concave posterior surface of an intervertebral disc is significant, perhaps even pathologic. Note that some epidural space is present at all levels between the posterior aspect of disc or vertebral body (Fig. 12.4);

this space is normally occupied by the posterior longitudinal ligament and anterior epidural veins.

EPIDURAL VEINS
AND ARTERIES

The draining veins of this region form a typical pattern, shown in Figure 12.2, and illustrated in Figure 12.3; the *basivertebral venous system* of a vertebral body communicates with (longitudinal) anterior and posterior *epidural veins,* which connect with external veins, then drain via the lumbar veins into the inferior vena cava.

The main arterial supply to the intradural structures is derived from radicular branches of the same arteries that supply the lumbosacral bony elements. The great radicular artery (of Adamkiewicz) supplies much of the lower spinal cord; it usually arises from the intercostal branches of the lower thoracic aorta, occasionally from the segmental lumbar arteries.

Large or engorged anterior epidural veins could suggest a bulging disc; however, their CT density is different from that of nucleus pulposus material. Moreover, intravenous contrast injections could clarify such a deformity (Fig. 12.5). The position of

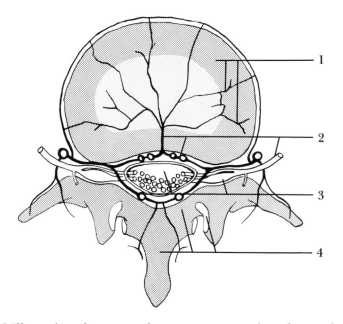

FIG. 12.3 Illustration of venous and nervous structures in and around a lumbar vertebra. *1,* Endplate, venous channels of body; *2,* basivertebral vein, anterior epidural veins, spinal nerve (ventral ramus); *3,* posterior epidural veins, dural sac with cauda equina, dorsal root ganglion; *4,* spinous process, lamina, superior articular facet. (Newton, T.H., and Potts, D.G. (eds.): Computed Tomography of the Spine and Spinal Cord. San Anselmo, Clavadel Press, 1983. Illustration modified from Chapter 4.)

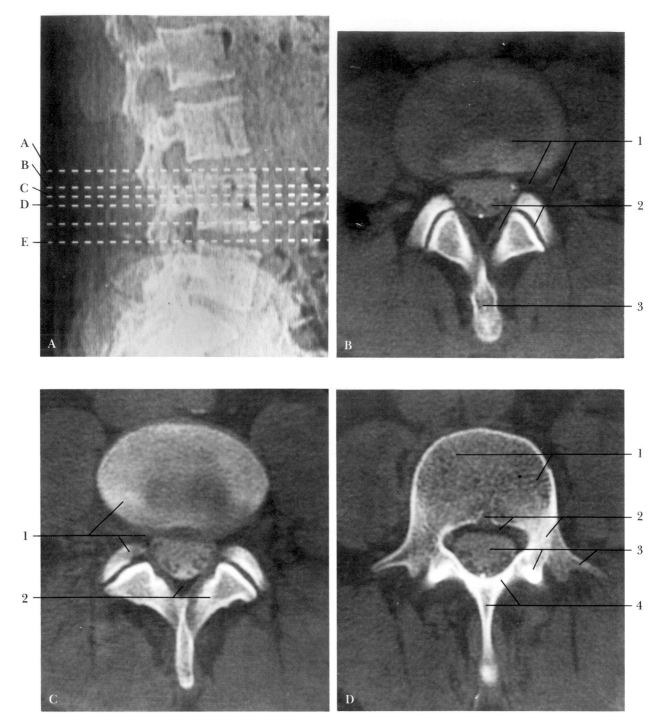

FIG. 12.4. Series of thin axial CT sections through lower lumbar vertebrae. **A.** Lateral scout view to indicate levels of sections. **B.** Level of L3/L4 disc. *1*, Disc, intervertebral foramen, dorsal root ganglion of L3; *2*, cauda equina, within dural sac, ligamentum flavum, facet joint; *3*, spinous process. **C.** Level of upper endplate of L4. *1*, Intervertebral foramen, superior articular process, endplate; *2*, lamina, epidural fat. **D.** Midbody of L4. *1*, Venous channels within body; *2*, opening for basivertebral vein, anterior epidural space, pedicle; *3*, dural sac, articular pillar, transverse process; *4*, spinous process, lamina.

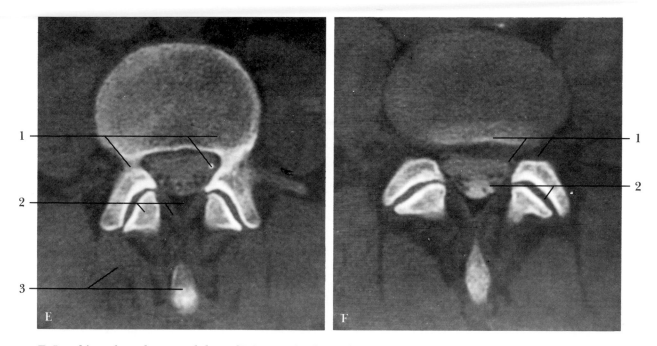

E. Level just above lower endplate of L4. *1*, Body, drop of Pantopaque, pedicle; *2*, epidural fat, ligamentum flavum, inferior articular process; *3*, spinous process, paraspinous musculature. **F.** Level of L4/L5 disc. *1*, Portion of endplate, nerve roots in lateral recess, intervertebral foramen; *2*, roots of cauda equina, facet joint space.

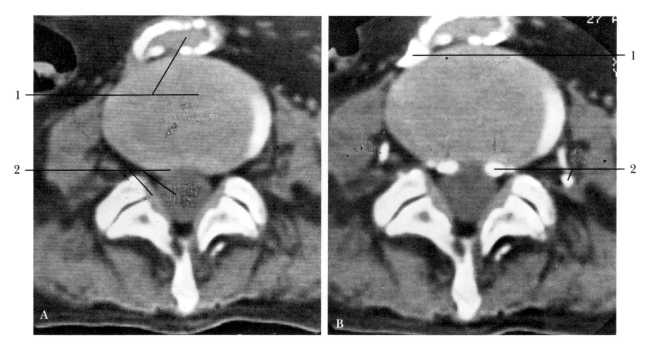

FIG. 12.5. CT images through L3/L4 disc, before and after venous contrast enhancement. **A.** Without contrast enhancement. *1*, disc, aorta with calcifications; *2*, anterior epidural vein, dural sac, ligamentum flavum. **B.** After intravenous contrast injection *1*, Inferior vena cava (partially filled); *2*, anterior epidural vein and ascending lumbar vein, both filled with contrast.

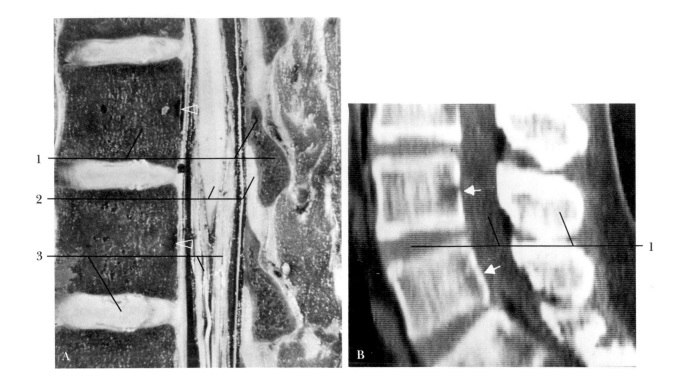

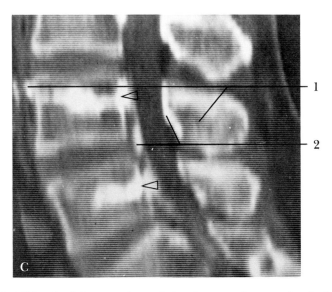

FIG. 12.6. Midsagittal images through lumbar vertebrae and spinal canal. **A.** Anatomic section: *1*, Transverse process, lamina, body of L3; *2*, ligamentum flavum, conus medullaris; *3*, cauda equina, nucleus pulposus. Anterior extradural space contains openings for basivertebral veins *(arrowheads)*. **B.** CT reformation without contrast enhancement. *1*, Nucleus pulposus of L3/L4 disc, vertebral canal, spinous process of L3 *(Arrows* indicate position of basivertebral veins). **C.** CT reformation after intravenous contrast. *1*, Anterolumbar vein, spinous process of L4; *2*, anterior epidural vein, posterior epidural vein *(Arrowheads* indicate basivertebral veins).

the basivertebral veins, emerging posteriorly at the midbody level, can be shown by midsagittal CT reformations and compared to an anatomic section (Fig. 12.6). The venous spaces within the vertebral body could theoretically be interpreted as fractures (Figs. 12.2C, 12.3, and 12.6).

High-resolution CT images may give adequate anatomic information regarding vertebrae and contents of the vertebral canal (Fig. 12.7). The outline of the *conus medullaris* with emerging nerve roots is visible in Figure 12.7A; the window settings in this image are not optimal for demonstrating the dural sac. The contour of the dural sac on CT images is determined by the surrounding low-density epidural fat; the nerve roots in the lateral recesses can sometimes be distinguished, as can the (anterior) epidural veins. Note that in Figure 12.7C the dural (thecal) sac has a posterior position within the vertebral canal; the prolonged, supine position of this particular patient led to displacement by gravity. Figure 12.7B represents a more normal position of the dural sac.

MORPHOLOGY OF THE SACRUM

The *sacrum* consists of five fused vertebrae with a continuous *sacral (vertebral) canal* and thin intervertebral discs (Fig. 12.8 and 12.9); the lower portion of the sacral canal opens as the *sacral hiatus* into the deep connective tissue of the posterior pelvic region. The termination of the dural sac (into a filum terminale externum) occurs normally at the S1 or S2 level. The spinous processes have fused to form a posterior median *sacral crest*. Pairs of anterior and posterior *sacral foramina* at each vertebral level permit passage of ventral and dorsal rami of the sacral nerves. The sacrum articulates with L5 and with the right and left ilium. A midsagittal MR image demonstrates not only the anterior concavity of the sacrum, but also the soft tissue structures and spaces in the pelvic region (Fig. 12.9).

SACROILIAC JOINT

The *sacroiliac joint* contains an anterior, smooth, diarthrodial portion, and a posterior, uneven, ligamentous portion (Fig. 12.8C). The diarthrodial surface is normally covered with a smooth lining of cartilage; the ligamentous portion forms the attachment for several strong ligaments (Fig. 12.8A). The normal appearance of the sacrum and sacroiliac joint on axial CT sections is not easy to interpret, unless the plane of section is adjusted to conform to the anatomic orientation of these structures. This can be done by tilting the gantry of the CT apparatus (up to 15°, after Carrera) or by changing the position of the patient be-

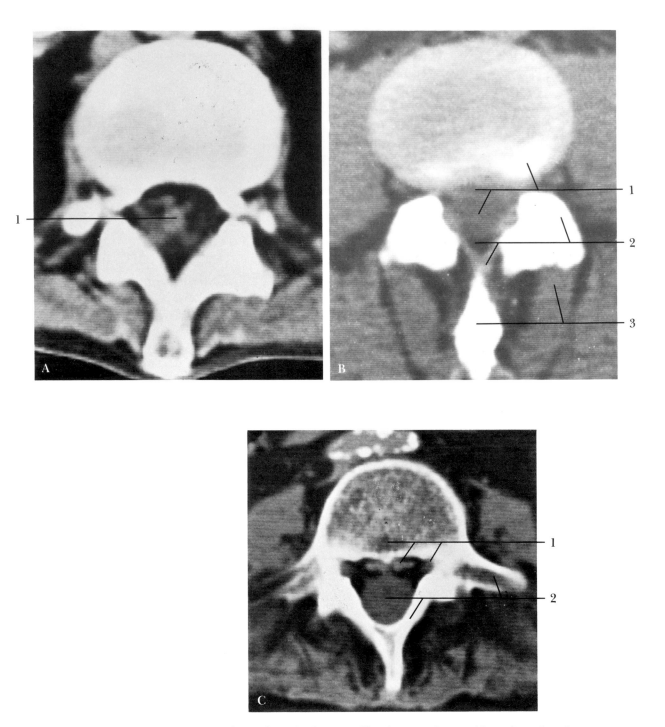

FIG. 12.7. Various CT images of lumbar vertebrae, without intrathecal contrast. **A.** Thick section at the level of L1. *1*, Conus medullaris with dorsal and ventral roots. **B.** Section at the level of upper endplate of L3. *1*, Epidural space, dural sac, endplate; *2*, epidural fat, ligamentum flavum, articular process; *3*, spinous process, paraspinous muscle. **C.** Thin section at the midbody level of L4. *1*, Basivertebral vein, anterior epidural vein, nerve roots in lateral recess; *2*, dural sac, lamina, transverse process.

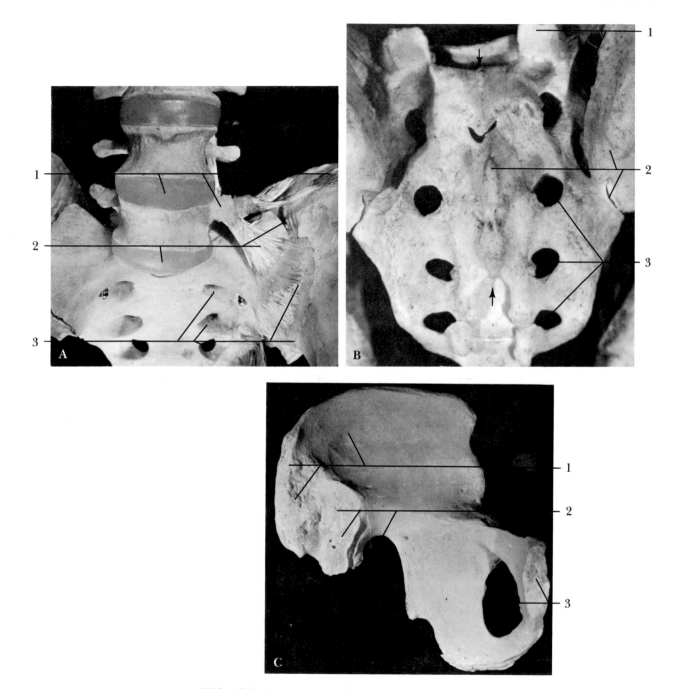

FIG. 12.8. Sacrum, sacroiliac joint, ligaments, and discs. **A.** Anterior view of lumbosacral region. *1*, Iliac crest transverse process of L5, L4/L5 disc; *2*, sacroiliac joint (ligamentous portion); lumbosacral ligament, L5/S1 disc; *3*, sacroiliac joint (diarthrodial portion), anterior sacral foramina. **B.** Posterior aspect. *1*, Superior articular facet of S1, sacroiliac joint (space for ligamentous portion); *2*, sacral crest, ilium, sacroiliac joint (diarthrodial portion); *3*, posterior sacral foramina. (*Arrows* indicate sacral canal at both ends.) **C.** Lateral aspect of left ilium. *1*, Sacroiliac joint (area for ligamentous portion), ilium; *2*, sacroiliac joint (diarthrodial portion), iliac notch; *3*, obturator foramen, pubic synostosis.

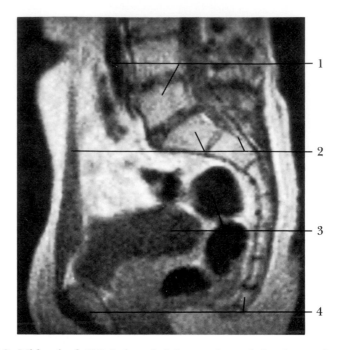

FIG. 12.9. Midsagittal MR (spin echo) image through lumbosacral region. *1*, Aorta, L5 body; *2*, rectus abdominis muscle, S1 body, end of dural sac; *3*, bladder, air in bowel; *4*, symphysis pubis, coccygeal vertebra.

fore scanning (Fig. 12.10A). Representative images of the diarthrodial and ligamentous portions of the sacroiliac joint are shown in Figure 12.10.

Altered Anatomy

The relationship between a cracked annulus fibrosus of an intervertebral disc, and a potential herniation of a fragment of the nucleus pulposus is shown in Figure 12.11; such a far lateral disc herniation cannot be demonstrated on a myelogram. Although CT images do not normally demonstrate details of the annulus fibrosus, a clinically significant herniation of a "disc" (nucleus pulposus) presumes lack of integrity of the annulus.

A traumatic "syrinx" in the thoracolumbar cord is shown in Figure 12.12. Such intramedullary cavities contain a fluid resembling CSF (hydromyelia), or blood in acute conditions (hematomyelia). The CT method can demonstrate a cavity by first injecting water-soluble contrast in the thecal sac, and then scanning after an interval of several hours. The contrast is transneurally absorbed into the syrinx. An MR image may directly demonstrate the syrinx fluid (which has a long T2) with a short echo delay (Fig. 12.12A). With a longer (second) echo delay,

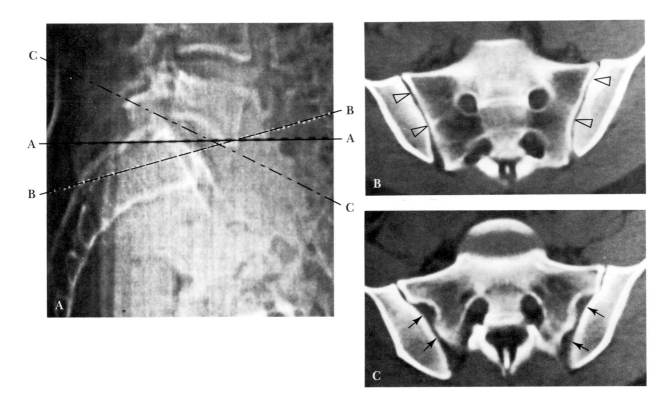

FIG. 12.10. CT images to illustrate sacroiliac joint (after Carrera and associates). **A.** Lateral scoutview. A-A normal axial plane; B-B optimal plane to demonstrate sacroiliac joint; C-C optimal plane to visualize L5/S1 disc. **B.** Image in B-B plane. Anterior, diarthrodial portions of sacroiliac joint *(arrowheads)*. **C.** Image parallel to B-B plane: posterior, ligamentous portion of sacroiliac joint *(arrows)*.

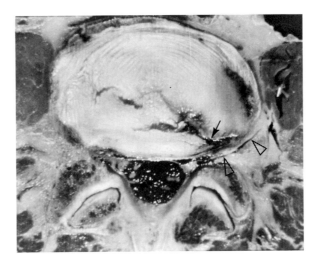

FIG. 12.11. Anatomic section through cracked L4/L5 disc. (compare with Figure 12.2A). An opening in the annulus fibrosus is present *(arrow)*, with disc material lateral to it *(arrowheads)*.

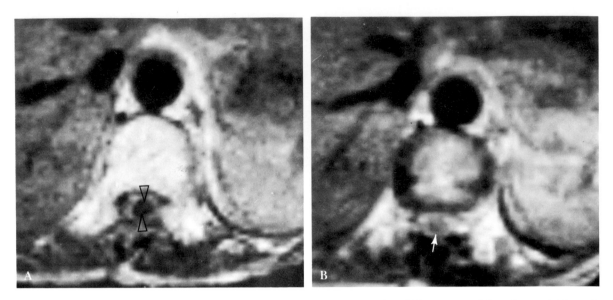

FIG. 12.12. Axial thoracolumbar MR images (spin echo) obtained with different repetition times. **A.** Repetition time is 0.5 sec. The vertebral canal is seen behind the vertebral body and aorta; a syrinx is present *(arrowheads)* within the cord. **B.** Repetition time is 2.0 sec. The syrinx *(arrow)* has a higher intensity signal (long T2 of the CSF-like fluid).

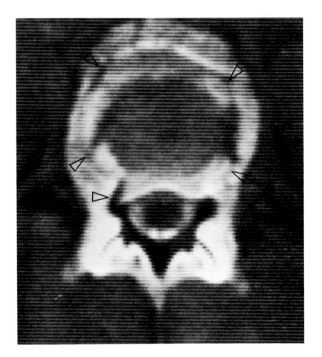

FIG. 12.13. Axial CT image with intrathecal contrast through upper L1 vertebral level. Numerous fractures are present *(arrowheads)*. (Federle, M.P., and Brant-Zawadski, M. (eds.): Computed Tomography in the Evaluation of Trauma. Baltimore, Williams & Wilkins, 1982.)

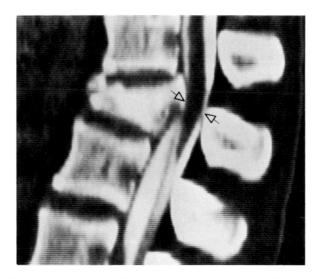

FIG. 12.14. Midsagittal reformation through lumbar spine of Figure 12.13. The body of L1 shows a compression fracture; the conus medullaris is compressed *(arrows)* between bone elements of L1. (Federle, M.P., and Brant-Zawadski, M. (eds.): Computed Tomography in the Evaluation of Trauma. Baltimore, Williams & Wilkins, 1982.)

the CSF-like fluid "fills in," and cannot be distinguished from the cord itself. The advantage of midsagittal CT reformations is shown in Figures 12.13 and 12.14; the axial images in Figure 12.13 (emergency scan of a patient who had fallen from a third floor window) show the presence of a compression fracture of the vertebral body. In the reformation (Fig. 12.14) the deformity of the vertebral column as a result of the collapsed vertebra is shown. The spinal cord appears compressed (which clinically was confirmed by the patient's paraparesis).

The intradural contrast used in the past was often slightly irritating to the nervous tissues, and therefore had to be removed after myelography. Remaining drops of contrast often caused a chemical arachnoiditis, resulting in chronic arachnoid adhesions often causing root-pain (Fig. 12.15; compare with Figs. 12.2B and 12.4E). The contrast used now is water-soluble and does not need to be removed since reabsorption occurs spontaneously.

An anatomic variant, often an incidental finding, is the so-called "conjoined" nerve root (Fig. 12.16). Although usually painless and infrequently present (an estimated incidence of less than 2%), this condition may resemble a lateral disc herniation on a myelogram; however, a careful evaluation of axial CT images made shortly after the myelogram explains the finding.

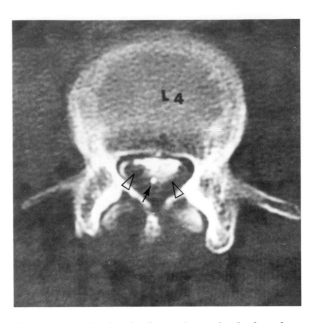

FIG. 12.15. CT image at L4 level of a patient who had undergone repeated myelography with Pantopaque. A drop of Pantopaque is seen *(arrow)*; the nerve roots of the cauda have become an adherent mass *(arrowheads)*.

An example of a congenital malformation in the lumbosacral region is a small lipoma of the filum terminale (Fig. 12.17); the low density of the mass (fat) aids in the diagnosis. This condition is often associated with a spina bifida with or without a meningocele (Fig. 12.18). The extent of the bulging dura, and its contents can be demonstrated best on CT with intrathecal contrast.

An excellent demonstration of the main landmarks and anatomic details of the lumbosacral region is given in Figure 12.19. These MR images demonstrate the normally occurring lumbar lordosis, especially in Figures 12.19C and 12.19D; the central region of each image represents a portion of the vertebral column which lies anterior to the top and bottom portions (see Figure 12.9).

Clinical Cases

CASE 22

A 42-year-old man sustained a minor injury to his low back area 2 months PTA while sliding in a baseball game at summer camp. Shortly thereafter, he noted dull pains in the lumbosacral region in the mornings. Three weeks PTA the patient felt the onset of sharp pain beginning in the R gluteal area and shooting down the back of his leg. This pain subsided after a day in bed;

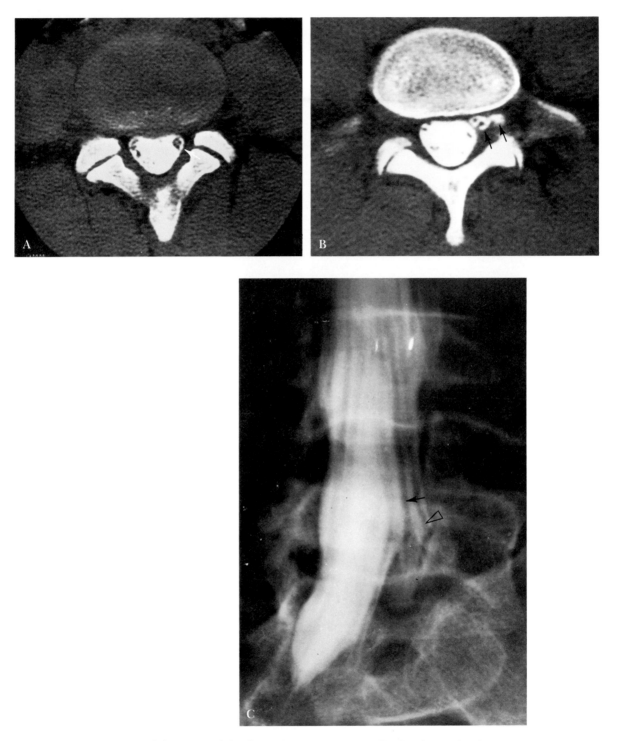

FIG. 12.16. Images pertaining to conjoined nerve roots. **A.** L4/L5 disc level. A pair of nerve roots is seen in the right lateral recess, while an aggregate of four nerve roots is seen in the left lateral recess *(arrow)*. **B.** Level of upper endplate of L5. Two nerve root sheaths are seen in the left intervertebral foramen *(arrows)*. **C.** Oblique lateral myelogram to show normal position of nerve root *(arrow)* and of conjoined nerve root *(arrowhead)*.

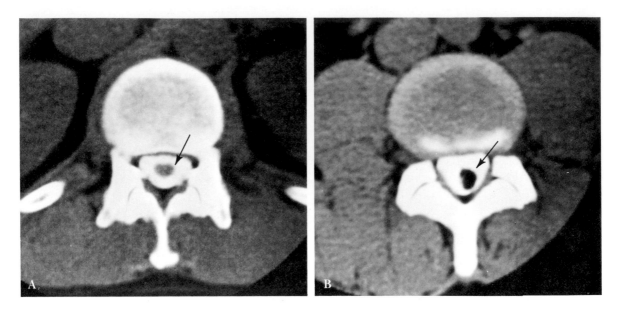

FIG. 12.17. CT images with intrathecal contrast in a child. **A.** The level of L1 shows a normal cord *(arrow)*. **B.** The level of the L3/L4 disc shows an enlarged filum terminale containing fat density *(arrow)*.

coughing, sneezing, straining, and bending precipitated an attack of pain again. The patient also noted occasional tingling of the R calf; he sometimes experienced back spasms.

NEX: MS: Intact. CNN: Intact.

Motor system: Strength intact.

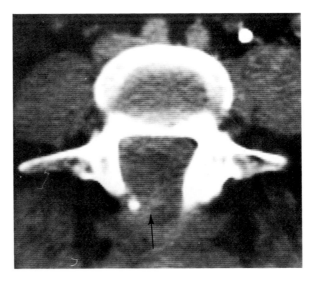

FIG. 12.18. CT image at the L5 endplate level. Note the absence of posterior elements *(arrow)* and large dural sac.

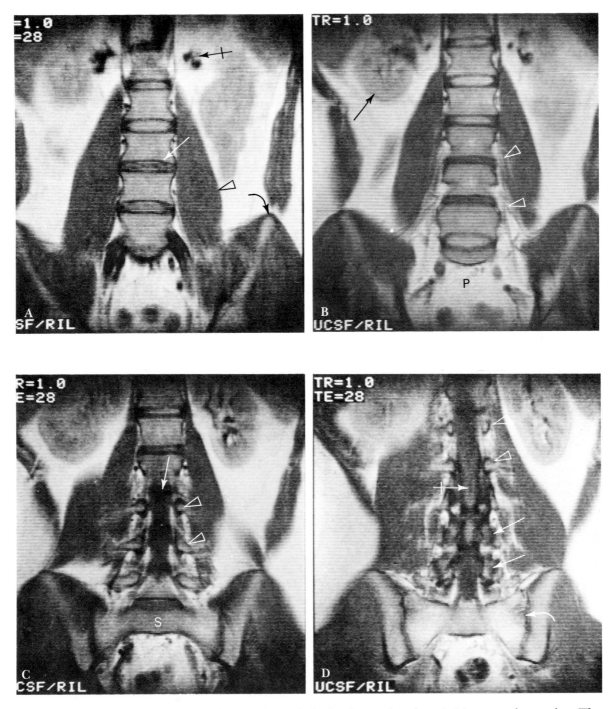

FIG. 12.19. Coronal MR (spin echo) images through the lumbosacral region. **A.** Most anterior section. The L3-4 intervertebral disc is minimally degenerated *(arrow)*; psoas muscle *(arrowhead)*, iliac crest *(curved arrow)* and contents of renal pelvis *(crossed arrow)* are clearly shown. **B.** Left kidney *(arrow)*, lumbar nerves *(arrowheads)*, and structures in the posterior pelvis (P) are visible. **C.** A column of CSF with L4 and L5 rootsleeves *(arrow)*, the pedicles of L3 and L4 *(arrowheads)* and the sacrum (S) are indicated. **D.** The pedicles of L1 and L2 *(arrowheads)*, facet joints of L4 and L5 *(arrows)*, and the sacroiliac joint *(curved arrow)* are seen. The contents of the dural sac are "averaged-in" with the laminae of L3 *(crossed arrow)* and L4.

DTRs: Intact in both UEs. R Achilles tendon reflex absent, normal L. R kneejerk slightly decreased. Plantar responses: flexor.

Sensory system: All modalities intact. Local pain on palpation of the sciatic nerve in the R buttock; local tenderness of L5/S1 area; marked spasm of the R paravertebral muscles. Straight leg raising limited to 30° on the R, normal on the L.

Lumbar spine films were normal. What other procedure would be helpful?

A CT study with intrathecal contrast was done (Fig. 12.20). What is your finding? What is your presumptive DX?

(Discussion of Case 22 and additional illustration on p. 217.)

CASE 23   A 42-year-old man complained of back pain, bladder problems, and impotence, all increasing over a 2-month period. His physician referred him to the neurologic service of a university hospital.

GPX: Well-developed, poorly nourished male, with an ulcer over both tubera ischii.

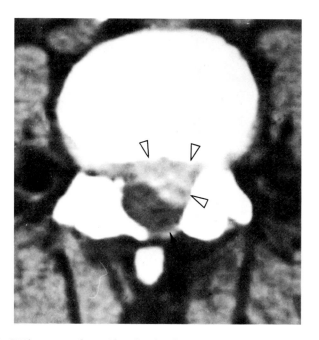

FIG. 12.20. CT image at the L4 level. The dural sac *(arrow)* has been compressed by a centrolateral large disc fragment *(arrowheads)*.

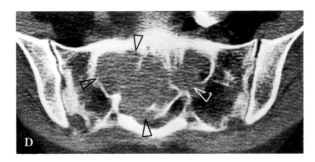

FIG. 12.21. CT image through the sacrum and sacroiliac joints. A large mass of intermediate density *(arrowheads)* has destroyed the normal configuration of the sacrum (see Figure 12.12).

NEX: MS: Depressed.

Motor system: Mild, flaccid paresis of both LEs, flexor muscles more than extensors. There was some atrophy in all leg muscles.

Sensory system: Loss of all sensation in perineal region and over the inner thighs.

An extensive radiologic study was done. Plain films over the lumbosacral region showed bone destruction of the sacrum and widening of the interpedicular space from L2 downwards. A CT scan was performed (Fig. 12.21). Your findings? Your DDX? (Discussion of Case 23 on p. 219.)

Questions

12a. A flattened posterior outline of the L3/L4 disc is seen on a CT image. Is this normal? If not, what could be the explanation of the finding?

12b. Which cord segments are contained in the conus medullaris? At which vertebral level does the conus normally end?

12c. What is the clinical importance of the basivertebral venous system?

12d. How can the components of the sacroiliac joint be examined best, using CT?

12e. How can the position of the end of the dural sac, its shape, and the possible presence of root cysts be determined?

12f. What are the possible locations of a herniated nucleus pulposus?

13. Discussion of 23 Cases

Case 1   Many people lose some of their mental sharpness and physical strength when they grow old; however, this patient was only in her early fifties when a decline in mental abilities was noted. During her stay in the hospital for an intercurrent disease (pneumonia) a neurologic exam was done: marked deficiencies in mental facilities, in muscular strength, and in coordination were seen. Pneumonia could explain the high leukocyte count. The patient's CT scan showed large ventricles, wide sulci, and an abnormally wide subarachnoid space for her age. The CT image (Fig. 2.18) is consistent with the generalized brain atrophy and enlargement of the CSF-spaces seen in much older people, often with little loss of mental or physical abilities. The patient's scan did not show localized abnormalities.

Based on the scan, history, and neurologic exam, the differential diagnosis would have to include the following: (pre)senile dementia with brain atrophy (possibly most marked in the frontal lobe), cerebral athero- or arteriolosclerosis, or rare diseases such as Huntington's chorea. The CSF findings in most of these would be within the normal range; EEG changes would be diffuse and nonspecific. Brain biopsy perhaps would result in the correct diagnosis but would not be indicated as there is no treatment for any of the possibilities mentioned.

The early age of onset and the absence of hypertension or other signs of vascular disease led to the diagnosis of *Alzheimer's disease* (senile dementia). There is no cure for this disease; the prognosis is poor (average survival, 5 years).

Case 2   This patient may show some signs of senile or pre-senile dementia (see Case 1); however, there are clear neurologic findings suggesting a frontal lobe lesion and involving at least the right precentral gyrus (seizure, paresis). The CT findings show a sharply defined round mass containing calcified areas with some reactive brain edema around it in the right hemisphere adjoining the skull; the mass is much denser after contrast enhancement.

The differential diagnosis includes tumor (slow-growing), abscess, bleeding. The last two can be ruled out by the history; the CT images are much more typical of a tumor than an abscess (see Fig. 3.14). The most prevalent type of hemispheric tumor with calcium at this age is a glioma; the peripheral location of the mass and the patient's gender are more compatible with a meningioma, which has a slower growth rate. External and internal carotid angiography could be useful in demonstrating the blood supply to this tumor, and in confirming the diagnosis; meningiomas have a rich supply from the external carotid artery, whereas gliomas do not.

The rapid deterioration of the patient was associated with beginning brain herniation (due to mass effect); an operation was done immediately. A *meningioma* was removed. The patient recovered quite well; there was marked improvement in most signs and symptoms. A careful examination of the scout view or digital radiograph (Fig. 13.1) demonstrates high-density areas that most likely represent calcium. An MR image of a proven meningioma in another patient demonstrates the surrounding edema quite

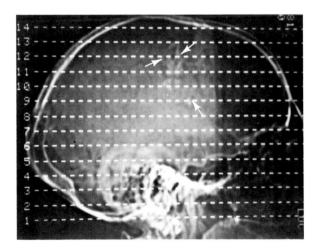

FIG. 13.1. The calcified areas of the tumor can be distinguished on the scout view *(arrows)*; line 11 represents the level of Figures 2.19A and B.

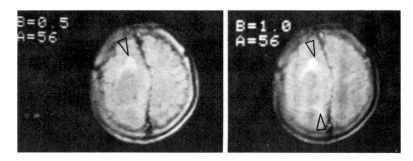

FIG. 13.2. Axial MR images (with different repetition times) at a level above the ventricles. A large low-signal mass is present, surrounded by high-signal zone with a long T2 (edema) best seen in the right image. There is mass effect.

well (Fig. 13.2); the high-intensity signal in the right image indicates a long T2, a finding compatible with edema.

Case 3 This patient's history indicates an increasingly frequent incidence of vertigo and headache; recently she had had a seizure, a sign of (motor) cortical irritation. Together with the papilledema, these signs and symptoms suggest increased cranial pressure, most likely due to a "mass." In the absence of signs of an infection such as an abscess or bleeding, a calcium-containing tumor must be suspected (shown by the skull film finding). The neuroradiologic procedures were essential for the precise localization of the mass, not for the diagnosis; the most frequently occurring tumor is a glioma.

Differential diagnosis includes abscess (see above), bleeding (hematoma, usually a sudden event), and acute hydrocephalus (could be secondary to a block in the CSF pathway). The tumor together with edema caused beginning brain herniation. The tumor, a *malignant astrocytoma*, proved to be inoperable, and its growth could not be controlled in time with drugs or radiation therapy.

Case 4 The history suggests that this aged man had had a fall (trauma) with a seizure afterwards (lip bite, incontinence). He was stuporous and mildly incapacitated when admitted, then grew steadily worse. There was no papilledema, which is an inconclusive finding at this time (it takes a day or so for papilledema to develop after a sustained and considerable increase in intracranial pressure). The sudden nature of this patient's severe problems after a relatively mild trauma suggests a *vascular event*. The small amount of blood in the CSF confirms this. (The use of lumbar puncture in making a diagnosis is now almost entirely restricted to cases with suspected infection of the meninges.) The CT scan shows a high-density zone (compatible with freshly clotted blood) high over the right hemisphere (Fig. 3.16).

This high-density zone could be a subdural hemorrhage, extradural hemorrhage, or even a subarachnoidal hemorrhage. The presence of blood within the CSF argues against an extradural hemorrhage. The findings that there is only a little amount of blood in the lumbar subarachnoid space, and that the bleeding is in a high location are not indicative of subarachnoidal bleeding; most subarachnoidal hemorrhages are caused by an aneurysm in large vessels at the base of the brain, or from an arteriovenous malformation anywhere in the brain.

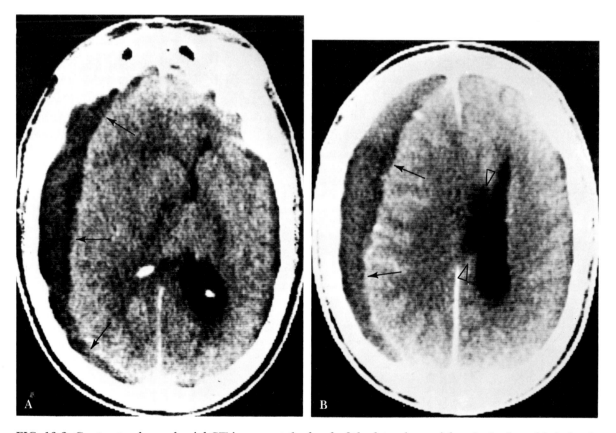

FIG. 13.3. Contrast-enhanced axial CT images at the level of the lateral ventricles. **A.** At the mid-thalamic level a large low-density area *(arrows)* is seen under the skull, causing a right to left shift; the right atrium is compressed. **B.** At the higher level the low-density area *(arrows)* has shifted the body of the right lateral ventricle across the midline *(arrowheads)*. The gyri of the right hemisphere appear to have a higher density than those on the left side; the effect is caused by compression and relative hyperperfusion.

This patient has suffered an *acute subdural hemorrhage*, caused by mild trauma, site of bleeding, atrophic brain (induced by age and alcohol) so that the bridging veins from brain to superior sagittal sinus are easily torn. Moreover, the unenhanced CT scan is quite typical: an extensive high-density mass compressing the brain high in the hemisphere; and an irregular medial outline conforming to the gyral pattern. The low-density area in Fig. 3.16B could be interpreted as renewed bleeding in progress.

The CT findings in another patient demonstrate a subdural mass, with a different density (Fig. 13.3). The patient has a similar history of mild trauma, sudden deterioration, and stupor, but in this case without brain herniation. The absence of blood density in the scan can be explained by the more chronic nature of the event: the patient's subdural hemorrhage occurred 7 months before the CT scan. When the blood had been resolved, a fluid-filled cavity (hygroma) remained. (Another more common cause of hygroma is cranial trauma, with tearing of the arachnoid and escape of CSF into the subdural space.)

Case 5   The patient presents a typical posttraumatic pattern: transient loss of consciousness, then a lucid interval, followed by increasing stupor (which may continue into coma and death). The patient's neurologic exam is within normal limits except for a possible abducens nerve paresis, and papilledema is not (yet) present. Vital signs are within normal limits. At this early stage the diagnosis is difficult to make without a CT scan; however, the patient should be observed regularly and carefully for signs of deterioration.

The differential diagnosis should include subarachnoidal hemorrhage from an aneurysm or arteriovenous malformation; epilepsy or seizure; systemic diseases associated with coma (e.g., diabetes mellitus, alcoholism, other intoxications) followed by trauma; and a sudden loss of consciousness from a heart attack or a severe intracranial hemorrhage from a torn blood vessel after trauma. High on the list is an extradural hemorrhage or a subdural hemorrhage. If time permits, a good differentiating procedure would be a blood test for sugar or alcohol levels; a lumbar puncture might be considered to diagnose a subarachnoid hemorrhage (see Case 10), but it is not without risk if a substantial intracranial bleeding is in progress (mass effect with herniation). The obvious diagnostic procedure was done here—an emergency CT scan (Fig. 4.17). This takes a short time (20 minutes or less)

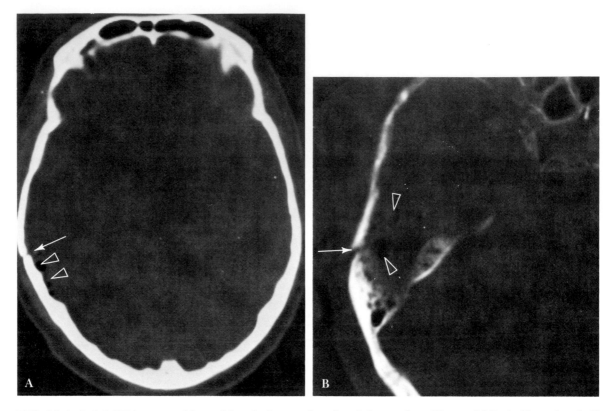

FIG. 13.4. Axial CT images with a wide window setting that is lower than Figure 4.17. **A.** Note the skull fracture *(arrow)* near the site of the extradural blood seen earlier. A few very low densities *(arrowheads)* are seen near the fracture. **B.** Lower (partial) CT image. The skull fracture *(arrow)* and the low-density areas *(arrowheads)* are again seen: air.

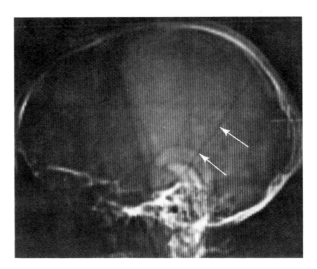

FIG. 13.5. The fracture *(arrows)* is clearly seen on a lateral scout view.

and demonstrates the location of the bleeding or bleedings, as well as an associated skull fracture (Fig. 13.4).

From the location of the bleeding (temporal bone area), its shape (lentiform), the skull fracture, and the typical history, the following diagnosis was made: *extradural hemorrhage* from a torn middle meningeal artery or branch. Moreover, the scout view (digital radiograph) demonstrates the fracture line (Fig. 13.5). This type of hemorrhage can be rapidly life-threatening (depending on the rate of bleeding) because it may cause herniation. The patient findings (rising blood pressure; lowered pulse rate and respiration rate) are suggestive of Cushing's phenomenon and indicate increasing pressure on the brain stem by beginning herniation.

Case 6 A sudden neurologic event has a vascular cause until proven otherwise. This patient has had a severe right-sided stroke affecting motor and sensory tracts above the foramen magnum, including the VIIth nerve pathway. The flaccidity of the left musculature is due to the abruptness of the event ("neural shock") and is also consistent with a hemorrhage in the internal capsule. The absence of papilledema is not significant since the formation of the intracranial mass has occurred quite recently.

In a middle-aged, hypertensive patient a stroke may be due to a subarachnoid hemorrhage from a ruptured aneurysm, a sudden occlusion of a large intracranial vessel, or an intracerebral hemorrhage. The CT scan aids in the diagnosis; a high-density mass in the region of the right lentiform nucleus, extending into the ventricles, represents an intracerebral bleeding with rupture into the ventricular system.

The diagnosis for this patient is typical: *hypertensive hemorrhage* from a ruptured lenticulostriate artery microaneurysm caused by long-standing high blood pressure.

Magnetic resonance images of an uncommon infarct in the region of the basal ganglia are shown in Figures 13.6 and 13.7. The inversion recovery image demonstrates the gray/white boundaries quite well; the lesion is visible. However, spin echo images with different repetition times and echo times are more diagnostic for the nature of the lesion.

Hypertensive hemorrhages tend to occur in a region where small vessels branch off from large diameter arterial trunks; most bleedings are found in the putamen-internal capsule (lenticulostriate arteries). Others occur in the thalamus (posterior perfora-

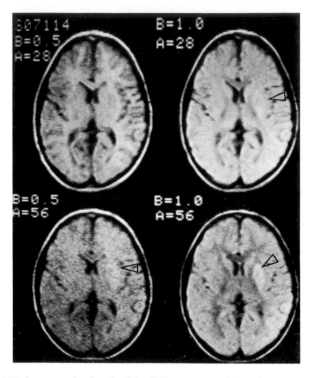

FIG. 13.6. MR images obtained with different repetition times and echo times. Note the varying high-intensity signal (infarct) in the left putamen *(arrowheads)*; the effect of a long T2 is best seen in the image with a long repetition time and a long echo time. Some mass effect is apparent in all images.

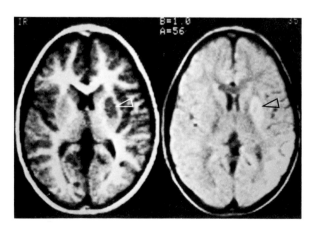

FIG. 13.7. MR images of the patient seen in Figure 13.6. (left, inversion recovery image; right, spin echo). A putaminal infarct is shown *(arrowheads)*.

tors; see Fig. 13.8); still others in the pons (pontine perforators) or in the cerebellum.

Case 7   The history in this patient suggests that a bronchial carcinoma has been removed, and that there may be metastases to neighboring areas since the spine film shows a lesion in the thoracic region. Intracranial metastases should therefore be included in the differential diagnosis. The principal and diverse neurologic signs (hemianopia, extraocular muscle movements, beginning papilledema, long motor tract signs) are all compatible with intracranial, multiple masses. Not surprisingly a CT scan (Fig. 5.14) was requested to aid in the localization of the lesions. The many high-density areas with surrounding edema are mostly situated in the vascular territory of the middle cerebral artery (which is common).

    Without the history, the CT images could be interpreted as multiple small abscesses, parasitic lesions, areas of demyelination,

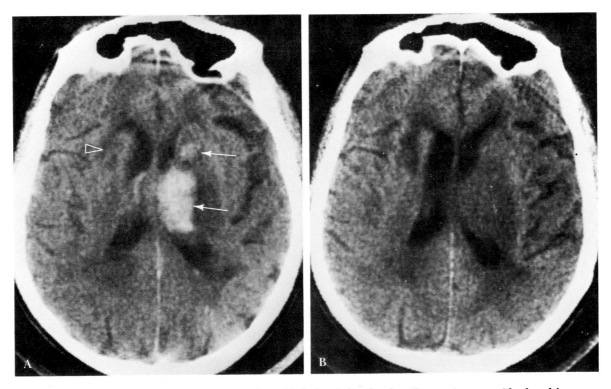

FIG. 13.8. Two unenhanced CT images at the mid-thalamic level, taken 6 months apart (the head is asymmetrically positioned). **A.** Two areas of high contrast are seen *(arrows)*; in an adjacent section these areas were shown to be continuous. There is a low-density area lateral to the right caudate nucleus *(arrowhead)*. **B.** The later scan shows resolution of the thalamic hemorrhage, although a slight mass effect remains. The infarct in the right caudate is still present.

or infarcts. However, the history indicates no infection or vascular problems; a parasitic infection tends to occur predominantly in patients from areas where parasites are common (not the case here). The patient's age is not indicative of a person with multiple sclerosis.

Most likely, the diagnosis is *brain metastases* secondary to lung cancer. The patient later died from an intercurrent pneumonia; he had been weakened by the underlying malignant process. Autopsy confirmed the presumptive diagnosis.

Case 8　Although the initial signs and symptoms, headache and nausea, are important in retrospect, they are not diagnostic; at best, a thought of a "mass" should be entertained. However, a more recent sign (inability to look up) is highly suggestive of a lesion in or near the vertical gaze center located in the pretectal region. The additional signs of papilledema complete the usual trio of symptoms for a mass (headache, nausea and vomiting, papilledema).

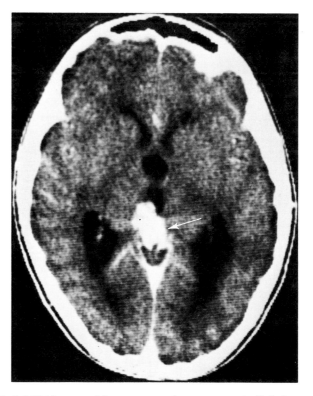

FIG. 13.9. Axial CT image with contrast enhancement. A slightly asymmetrical, irregular, high-density mass *(arrow)* behind the third ventricle is present; the ventricles are enlarged.

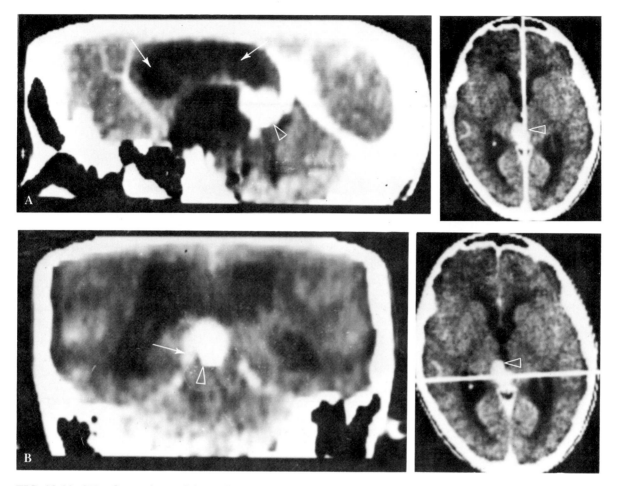

FIG. 13.10. CT reformations of the series of scans represented by Figure 13.9; the planes of reformation are indicated on axial scans. **A.** Sagittal image. Note the low-density third ventricle behind the anterior cerebral artery; the lateral ventricle appears enlarged *(arrows)*. There is a high-density mass *(arrowhead)* between third ventricle and cerebellar apex. **B.** Coronal image. Note the high-density mass *(arrowhead)* below the apex of the tentorium *(arrow)*; the enlarged lateral ventricles are clearly seen.

The CT scan (Fig. 5.15) shows an enhancing mass in midline, between the posterior thalami, most likely involving the pineal gland.

The diagnosis was *pineal region tumor.* Such neoplasms are not common (1% of all brain tumors). There are three main types: pineal teratoma, pinealoblastoma, and pinealocytoma. The first type is more common, grows rapidly, and may seed; it occurs mainly in young men. Sometimes the tumor grows posteriorly (rather than anteriorly as in our Case 8); then cerebellar signs begin to occur, as well as signs and symptoms of a posterior fossa mass (ataxia, loss of vertical and some lateral gaze, nystagmus, and decreased hearing).

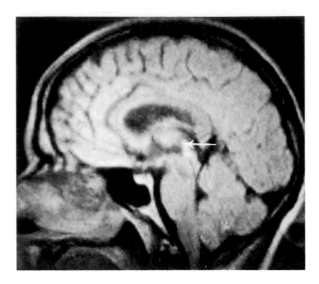

FIG. 13.11. Direct midsagittal MR image (compare with Figure 5.9 and Fig. 13.10A). A small high-signal mass *(arrow)* is present above the superior colliculus.

Compression of the aqueduct and subsequent noncommunicating hydrocephalus occur in most patients with pineal tumors of some size. Figures 13.9 and 13.10 demonstrate the usefulness of reformations in addition to the axial scan. The diagnosis was a pineal tumor. A direct, sagittal MR image shows another tumor in the pineal region with some degree of hydrocephalus (Fig. 13.11). This tumor was a germinoma, a form of teratoma.

Case 9   The patient's history of transient ischemic attacks is highly suggestive of cranial atherosclerotic, occlusive vessel disease. A transient ischemic attack is sometimes referred to as reversible ischemic neurologic deficit (RIND); it can be followed by a full-blown stroke. The carotid bruit suggests the presence of stenosis. An angiographic study of the neck vessels or the cerebral arteries, or both, may yield much information; a venous digital subtraction angiogram is the safest method. Computed tomography scanning cannot make the diagnosis unless occlusion of a branch of a vessel or the vessel itself has occurred.

Figure 6.20 can only be interpreted as total occlusion of the middle cerebral artery. The extent of low density is typical for the territory of the middle cerebral artery. Note in the scan that the thalamus, supplied by the perforators of the basilar/posterior cerebral artery complex, has escaped damage. The diagnosis, therefore, is a *total infarct of the middle cerebral artery,* preceded by transient episodes of circulation deficiency caused by spasms or resolving emboli from more proximal atheromatous sources.

Another, milder case is shown in Figure 13.12A. The low densities are in the middle cerebral artery distribution; the diagnosis is occlusion of branches of the middle cerebral artery. Figure 13.12B shows at least two.

In the past, angiography was the only procedure able to demonstrate the extent of a vascular occlusion or stenosis. Abrupt occlusion of a major vessel is more likely to occur without the formation of anastomotic channels (Fig. 13.13). Gradual occlusion may show a revascularization from other sources, so that the functional deficit is less severe.

Case 10   This patient shows a combination of symptoms: a sudden, severe headache; stupor; and, later, loss of consciousness. These symptoms, along with the patient's history of hypertension and

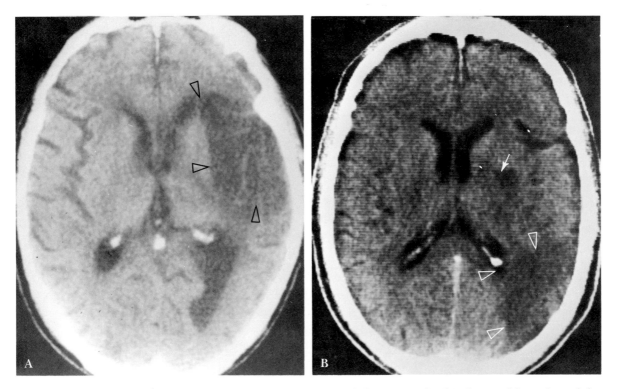

FIG. 13.12. CT images without contrast enhancement. **A.** An infarct *(arrowheads)* of several branches of the middle cerebral artery is seen in the left hemisphere. **B.** (Different patient) An infarct *(arrow)* is present in the left putamen; a large, wedge-shaped infarct *(arrowheads)* is seen in the left parietal lobe.

neurological signs, indicate a vascular event. The neck stiffness (meningeal irritation) suggests the presence of blood in the lower cisterns in the absence of signs of an infectious process such as meningitis. In the years before CT was developed, lumbar puncture would have shown frank blood in the CSF.

Of the possible vascular lesions in the CNS, a possible subarachnoid hemorrhage should be high on the list of differential diagnoses; an occlusion of a major vessel is not likely since there is indirect evidence of a bleeding. An intracranial hemorrhage with extension into the CSF spaces should also be considered. A diagnostic angiogram in the acute stage, and even a digital angiogram are contraindicated; the diagnostic method of choice is a CT scan *without contrast,* to show the pattern of high density (blood) in the cisterns or brain (Fig. 6.22).

On the basis of the history and examination, as well as the scan, the diagnosis of *subarachnoid hemorrhage* was made: the blood density is entirely restricted to the basal cisterns. Such a subarachnoid hemorrhage may be caused by the rupture of an aneurysm, leakage, or rupture of the vessels of an arteriovenous malformation. Sometimes the distribution of blood suggests the site of bleeding; sometimes the aneurysm itself may be visible by its size or calcification. Once the acute attack has subsided an angiogram is done to give the neurosurgeon more precise information regarding the origin of the bleeding.

Case 11   The symptoms that developed first were headaches (nonspecific complaint) and decreased vision. The localization of the lesion along the visual pathway is aided by the finding of a bitemporal hemianopia, which indicates that the problem exists in or near the chiasma. The headaches plus the flat optic discs (perhaps beginning papilledema) suggest an intracranial mass.

A mass in the chiasma region has a long list of possibilities: large pituitary tumor (typically with a bitemporal hemianopia and endocrine disturbances); craniopharyngioma (a tumor that lies often high in or above the sella); aneurysm of a vessel in the suprasellar cistern; glioma of the chiasma itself; tumor (e.g., glioma) of the frontal region; or an aneurysm of the anterior communicating artery. A further diagnostic study is clearly indicated.

The CT scan (Fig. 6.22) shows a partially enhancing mass above the chiasma, in the region of the anterior cerebral vessels (the reformations are particularly helpful). An angiogram was done because the diagnosis of aneurysm was likely (in Fig. 13.14

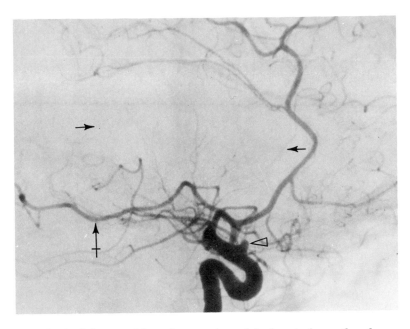

FIG. 13.13. A right carotid angiogram (arterial phase) shows the absence of contrast in the territory of the middle cerebral artery *(arrows)*; a small aneurysm is seen at the origin of the ophthalmic artery *(arrowhead)*; the posterior cerebral artery *(crossed arrow)* is filled from the internal carotid artery.

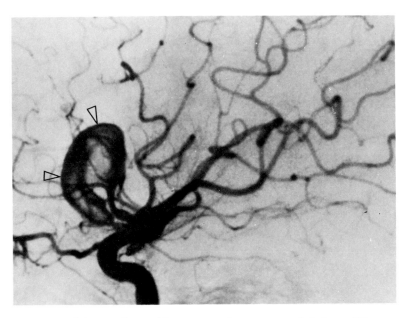

FIG. 13.14. Left internal carotid artery angiogram, arterial phase. The mass of Figure 6.23 is shown to be a partially thrombosed aneurysm *(arrowheads)*, probably of the anterior communicating artery.

the aneurysm is seen as a round, partially vascular mass close to a vessel). The diagnosis of a *partially thrombosed aneurysm of the anterior communicating artery* was made. Such "giant aneurysms" are often partially thrombosed, sometimes have a rim of calcification, and "behave" as a mass. (The slightly increased deep tendon reflexes could not be explained by the aneurysm.) The aneurysm was successfully removed, and the headaches and visual problems disappeared.

Case 12   A gradual increase of signs and symptoms over a period of months indicates the presence of a growing mass within the cranial cavity. In this case, the bitemporal hemianopia together with hormonal deficiencies suggest a pituitary tumor with suprasellar extension.

   In addition the differential diagnosis would have to include a craniopharyngioma (usually cystic and partially calcified), rare hypothalamic tumors, and possibly other conditions in the sellar region (Cushing's disease, Rathke's pouch cyst, rarely with visual symptoms). The vital signs are in the low-normal range, consistent with thyroid dysfunction or lack of secretion of thyroid stimulating hormone.

   The CT scan (Fig. 7.14) is useful because it rules the other possibilities out; however, the precise histologic nature of the *pituitary tumor* mass cannot be identified with certainty. The dark cross on the axial scans is a beam-hardening artifact due to the presence of dense bone in that plane, usually the petrous pyramids. This dense bone degrades both the initial scan and the derived reformations. It can be avoided by changing the plane of scanning with the help of the lateral scout view.

   A large pituitary adenoma, mainly growing down into the sphenoid sinus, is seen in Figure 13.15A. Another patient is shown in Figure 13.15B; there were no endocrinologic signs whatsoever. It was assumed that the low-signal mass in the pituitary represented a pars intermedia cyst.

Case 13   As with the patient in Case 11, a combination of headache and especially visual problems suggests a lesion in the patient's visual pathway. Additionally, the reduction in libido (provided it is not due to psychological problems) points to the hypothalamus or the pituitary gland. A further neurodiagnostic procedure is indicated to give insights as to the location and size of the lesion

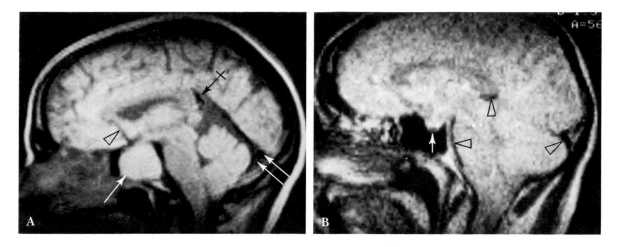

FIG. 13.15. Direct sagittal MR images (spin echo). **A.** A large high-intensity signal area *(arrow)* represents a pituitary adenoma. Note the anterior cerebral artery *(arrowhead)*, great vein *(crossed arrow)*, confluence *(double arrow)*, red nucleus, and inferior olivary nucleus in the brain stem. **B.** (Different patient) Second echo. A small low-density area *(arrow)* represents a pars intermedia cyst. The great vein, confluence, and basilar artery are clearly visible *(arrowheads)*.

(Fig. 7.14). The CT scan makes it clear that a mass is present below the chiasma. The differential diagnosis therefore is pituitary tumor (the scan indicates a tumor above a flattened gland); a craniopharyngioma (a tumor that may be intrasellar or above the diaphragma sellae), or a rare hypothalamic tumor. The presumptive diagnosis was *craniopharyngioma,* mainly because the visual problems became manifest first. The diagnosis was confirmed after neurosurgical removal of the mass.

This type of tumor may occur at any age, although there is a higher incidence in the prepubertal period and in late adulthood. A smaller tumor located clearly above the diaphragma is seen in Figure 13.16. Cyst formation, a calcium deposit in or on the rim of the tumor, is common, as seen in Figure 13.17.

Case 14 This young patient has the essential signs and symptoms of an intracranial mass: headache, papilledema, and nausea and vomiting. The time course is in agreement with that assumption. The cerebellar signs, the spontaneous nystagmus, and the long tract signs suggest a posterior fossa lesion, probably in the cerebellum, or in the brain stem with interruption of cerebellar pathways. The latter is unlikely because of the limited long tract signs, and the absence of cranial nerve signs, except of the vestibular nerve (which has connections with the archicerebellum).

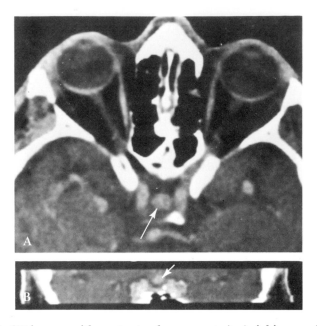

FIG. 13.16. CT images with contrast enhancement. **A.** Axial image. An enhancing mass *(arrow)* is seen between the internal carotid arteries. **B.** The coronal reformation shows the mass *(arrow)* in the suprasellar cistern.

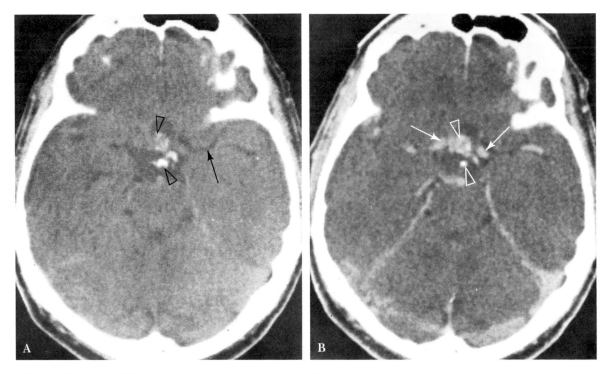

FIG. 13.17. Axial CT images. **A.** An irregularly calcified mass *(arrowheads)* is visible in the suprasellar cistern. Note the position of the middle cerebral artery *(arrow)*. **B.** Image with contrast enhancement. The calcified mass *(arrowheads)* is seen between the internal carotid arteries *(arrows)*.

The findings of the complete blood count and the absence of neck stiffness rule out an infectious process. A CT study would be useful; however, a CT cisternogram would not only show the location of the mass (pons or cerebellum, or both) but also whether the mass is intra- or extra-axial. The result of the CT scan (Fig. 8.19) shows a relatively normal supratentorial compartment and a low density in the posterior fossa compressing the fourth ventricle. How should these findings be put together? The commonest posterior fossa tumors in children are medulloblastoma (solid, growing down from the cerebellar vermis, often seeding), ependymoma (solid, usually growing on the floor of the fourth ventricle), and glioma (especially the cystic type in the cerebellum), or the solid pontine glioma.

The diagnosis is *cystic astrocytoma with a mural nodule*. The nodule is visible on Figure 8.19B as a small, high-density mass in the lateral cerebellum.

Case 15   As with the patient in Case 14, the signs and symptoms of an intracranial mass in the posterior fossa are present in this patient. In this case, the cerebellar signs are less severe, and the long tract and cranial nerve signs more pronounced. The CT scan and especially the reformation is diagnostic (Fig. 8.20).

The only diagnosis that fits the signs and symptoms in this age group, and with this scan, is a *pontine glioma*.

In another case, a direct MR scan was done (Fig. 13.18). Here the location is clearly shown, but also the nature of the pontine mass, which is partially cystic, partially hemorrhagic, partially solid; there are no posterior fossa artifacts.

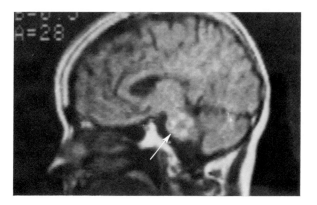

FIG. 13.18. Direct sagittal MR image (spin echo). The pontine lesion *(arrow)* contains high-signal areas (slow-flowing blood or post-radiation changes) and a low-intensity center (cystic necrosis).

Case 16   This patient demonstrates the typical signs of hyperthyroidism: exophthalmos, tremor, weakness of eye and body muscles (Graves' disease). The CT scan shows a mild protrusion of the right eye and a striking increase in the size of certain extraocular muscles, especially the lateral rectus on both sides (Figs. 9.14 and 9.15). The reformations are most useful in demonstrating the difference in size between similar muscles in the two eyes. The findings are typical and confirmatory of the diagnosis of *Graves' disease*.

Case 17   The infectious nature of the disease is suggested by the patient's history: acne and severe nasal infection with signs of systemic spreading. The differential diagnosis therefore is limited; infectious processes in the orbit are pseudotumor, adenitis of the lacrymal gland, angiitis with or without thrombosis, systemic infections. The CT scan in this patient is rather typical (Figs. 9.16 and 9.17).

A diagnosis of *infectious thromboangiitis* of the superior ophthalmic vein was made, mainly based on the patient's history, physical examination, and the ophthalmologic examination; the CT scan confirmed the diagnosis.

Case 18   The familial history of this patient, his age, and the physical findings suggest an intracranial congenital condition associated with dilated ventricles, cortical irritation (pressure?), and long motor tract signs.

Malformations in the central nervous system (CNS) in which obstructive hydrocephalus is present include aqueductal stenosis (rarely causing hemiparesis); Dandy-Walker syndrome (membranous closure of fourth ventricle, absence of vermis), and a form of Chiari malformation. The CT scan (Fig. 10.17) is diagnostic, provided the size of the fourth ventricle can be assessed: it is normal in aqueductal stenosis; large in Dandy-Walker syndrome; normal or small in Chiari malformation with tonsillar herniation. A midsagittal reformation is especially useful for diagnosis (Fig. 13.19A).

There are at least three forms of the Chiari malformation; the Chiari I type is the least complex. The Chiari II type, which includes the presence of a meningocele, is referred to as Arnold-Chiari malformation. This case represents the *Chiari II type;* it may include an enlarged foramen magnum, tonsillar herniation,

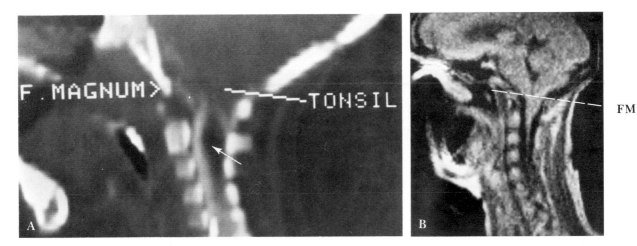

FIG. 13.19. Parasagittal images. **A.** CT reformation of the patient in Case 18. The cerebellar tonsil protrudes below the large foramen magnum; the upper cord shadow *(arrow)* is larger than normal. **B.** Direct MR image (first echo). The cerebellum extends below the level of the foramen magnum *(FM)*.

"buckling" of the cervical cord, medullary herniation, and flattening or "beaking" of the quadrigeminal bodies. Other malformations may be present (spina bifida, syringomyelia, skull abnormalities).

The anatomic relationships around the foramen magnum can be directly visualized in (para)sagittal planes with the MR imaging method. Figure 13.19B demonstrates another Chiari malformation in a 3-year-old girl; at the time of scanning she was in reasonably good health, unlike the boy discussed earlier in Case 18.

Case 19   This case is difficult at first because a part of the history was not given during the first interview with the patient. The spine films showed a minimal subluxation in the C-spine; the patient, when questioned further, said that the weakness began soon after a diving accident in which she hit the bottom of the swimming pool. Now the link between the trauma to the spine and progressive spinal cord disease is clearer, and the localization of the lesion is suggested by the plain spine film.

The combination of loss of pain and temperature sense, motor tract signs, and hyperhidrosis suggests a large central cord lesion involving several long tracts including the descending sympathetic pathway. The thick speech (dysarthria) indicated that the process had progressed to involve nuclei in the medulla (cranial nerve XII, probably). The CT scan confirms this involvement (Fig. 10.18).

The diagnosis is *traumatic syringomyelia and syringobulbia*. Such cavities in the neuraxis may occur after relatively mild trauma, although usually the trauma is more severe. In most cases the syrinx enlarges longitudinally, frequently upwards (as in this case).

Case 20   The history suggests a neurologic process in the lower cervical cord. Sudden pain when coughing or sneezing is a sign of dorsal root compression (in this case on the left side). The decreased biceps and radial reflexes are compatible with peripheral nerve lesions at the C6 level. The long tract signs are limited to the descending motor system and the spinothalamic pathway. There is a loss of sensation in the area of the C6 and C7 levels.

A compression of the cord at the level of the root signs is likely. This combination of signs and symptoms could be due to a nerve root tumor (schwannoma or neurofibroma), a meningioma, a herniated nucleus pulposus, spondylosis with narrowing of the vertebral canal and intervertebral foramina. The patient's history is somewhat confusing and is not typical for a tumor. In any case, a further neurodiagnostic examination appeared indicated.

On the basis of the appearance, density, and location of the mass on a CT scan (Fig. 11.16) the diagnosis of centrolateral *hernia nuclei pulposi* was made. The MR imaging method is similarly useful in documenting space-occupying lesions (Fig. 13.20).

Case 21   It is assumed that there are no cranial nerve deficits, and that there are no indications that the cerebellum or cerebrum is involved. In contrast to Case 20, the signs and symptoms in this patient indicate a lesion that is primarily intradural, probably intramedullary: there are several long tract signs, and the sensory systems are extensively involved. The side of the lesion is suggested by the preponderance of the left-sided motor signs and the right-sided loss of pain sense (indicative of a crossed spinothalamic tract); the *level* of the lesion is indicated by the wrist drop and triceps atrophy (C7/C8).

The differential diagnosis should include syringomyelia (the one-sided pain loss and lack of trauma in the patient's history does not suggest this diagnosis); an intramedullary tumor, and multiple sclerosis of the cord (the patient's age and the lack of

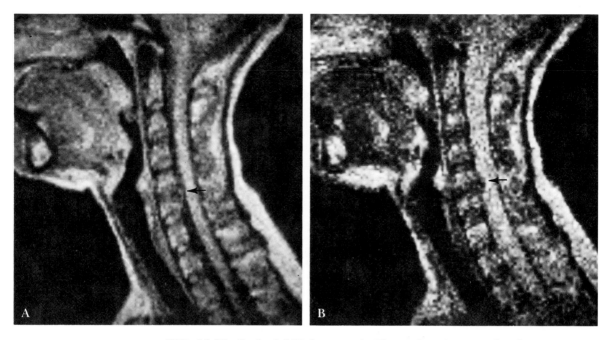

FIG. 13.20. Sagittal MR images. **A.** First echo. An extradural mass *(arrow)* protrudes into the clearly visible CSF column at the C5/C6 level. **B.** Second echo. The CSF (long T2) now has a high signal, so that the disc protrusion *(arrow)* stands out.

signs and symptoms above the foramen magnum make this diagnosis unlikely). The CT scan was useful in demonstrating an enlarged cord, making the correct diagnosis clearer.

An intrinsic, *intramedullary cord tumor* at this level could be an ependymoma, a glioma, or, rarely, hemangioblastoma. The histologic diagnosis, a glioma, could only be made postoperatively. The tumor was almost completely removed with the help of laser microsurgery; there were residual neurologic deficits.

A sagittal CT reformation (not shown in this book) was useful to the neurosurgeon by showing the longitudinal extent of the cord tumor. A direct MR image in another patient (Fig. 13.21) demonstrates the presence of an abnormal cord enlargement equally well (or better). In this case the intramedullary tumor was an ependymoma.

Case 22   The patient's history, a sudden sciatica-like pain in the lower back, aggravated by coughing, sneezing, straining, etc., is highly suggestive of abrupt pressure on a sensory root. Increase in intra-abdominal pressure increases the pressure within the dural sac and causes swelling of the veins, e.g., in the intervertebral canal (see Fig. 12.3), and the pain becomes suddenly worse.

The differential diagnosis should include herniated nucleus pulposus ("slipped disc"), a traumatic stenosis of the vertebral canal, or a loose fragment from a herniated disc elsewhere.

The most common condition with these symptoms is *hernia nuclei pulposi*. The history and physical examination helped determine the probable level (L5/S1), on the left side. This condition was confirmed by a CT scan at that level (Fig. 12.19). Such centrolateral "discs" may be visible on a myelogram including several views; a far-lateral disc cannot be demonstrated by myelography. The combination of intrathecal contrast in the dural sac and a CT scan is at present the diagnostic method of choice. Plain films of the lower vertebral column do not indicate the herniation itself; however, the decreased height of the intervertebral disc is suggestive of herniation. The MR imaging method can demonstrate a lumbar hernia nuclei pulposi, although the resolution is not yet as good as CT (Fig. 13.22).

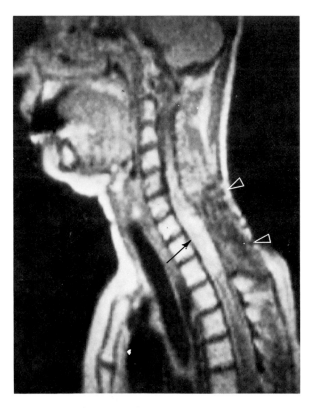

FIG. 13.21. Sagittal MR image (spin echo) of a recurrent ependymoma. The cord is enlarged between C5 and T3 *(arrow)*; a postoperative defect *(arrowheads)* is visible. The anatomic details of the sternum, trachea, and vertebral column are clearly seen.

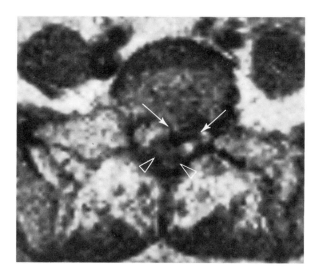

FIG. 13.22. Axial MR image (spin echo) at the level of L5/S1. Compare with Figures 12.2 and 12.19. A partially calcified, centrolateral disc herniation *(arrows)* compresses the dural sac *(arrowheads)*; the high-intensity epidural fat is asymmetrically present. The psoas muscles, iliac vessel, and sacroiliac joints are visible (not labeled).

Case 23   The history indicates a lesion in the lower spinal column. The flaccid paresis of the lower extremities and the atrophy in the leg muscles indicate a lower motor neuron lesion in the conus or in the cauda equina. The loss of sensation in the lower lumbar and sacral regions confirms that the neurologic deficit is extensive and involves the entire lower cord or the cauda, or both. The radiologic studies are highly suggestive of a destructive tumor in the lower spine region.

The differential diagnosis should include not only intrinsic cord tumors, but also root tumors, bone tumors, or infection (the patient's history makes the latter very unlikely). On the strength of the CT scan (Fig. 12.20) a presumptive diagnosis of *spinal cord tumor* was made; the most frequent neoplasm in this region is an *ependymoma*. This was confirmed by a biopsy. The inoperable tumor continued to grow despite radiation and chemotherapy; the patient died 9 months after the first scan was made.

14. Answers to Questions

Chapter 2

2a. The CT density of bone is in the order of 800 to 1000 Hounsfield units for compact bone; diploic bone is much lower (100 to 500 Hounsfield units), while bone containing air cells, such as the mastoid, has irregular areas of very low density. The CT density of CSF is 0 to 16 Hounsfield units, and is somewhat dependent on protein content (highest in the lumbosacral subarachnoid space).

2b. The CT density of white matter is less (24 to 36 Hounsfield units) than that of gray matter (32 to 50 Hounsfield units); the difference is more pronounced after contrast enhancement.

2c. Skull bones can be visualized in sharp detail if very wide windows are used, e.g. 2,000 or 4,000 units (Extended Scale and ReView, special General Electric computer programs), in thin sections.

2d. The falx and the tentorium can be seen better after contrast enhancement, due to the absence of a blood-brain barrier in these structures, and the presence of capillaries.

2e. The MR imaging signals in the inversion recovery mode are lower for gray matter than for white matter; thus, a more "natural" image is obtained.

2f. The cortex contains relatively more small blood vessels; hence its better visibility after (intravenous) contrast injection.

2g. The infraorbitomeatal base plane passes through the lower rims of the orbits and the external auditory meatuses.

2h. The tip of the anterior (frontal) horn lies slightly lower than the interventricular foramen (Monro's foramen, see Fig. 2.4).

2i. Normally, the first cut is taken through the foramen magnum; the last one ideally includes the top of the skull, especially if abnormalities are suspected there (e.g., meningioma of the falx, superior sagittal sinus thrombosis, etc.)

2j. The cortex of the precentral gyrus is almost twice as wide as that of the postcentral gyrus (see Figs. 2.8 and 2.9).

2k. Structures that do not possess a blood-brain barrier become more CT dense after contrast enhancement, so that abnormal elements without such a barrier (tumors, infectious masses, etc.) stand out more clearly.

Chapter 3 3a. The choroid plexus cannot be demonstrated in the anterior horn because the plexus does not extend in front of the interventricular foramen.

3b. The splenium contains visual associative fiber systems.

3c. Images of the genu and the splenium can be readily obtained with CT; the body and the callosal radiations are less clearly seen as a rule in horizontal (axial) sections.

3d. At least three lobes are seen at the level of section B: the frontal, the parietal, and the superior gyrus of the temporal lobe; the insula and the upper portion of the occipital lobe may also be included in thick sections at this level.

3e. The falx, a curved structure, in Section B is cut in two places: anteriorly and posteriorly, close to its junction with the tentorium (see Figs. 2.2, 2.5, and 2.6).

3f. The choroid plexus does not have a blood-brain barrier, as can be demonstrated by its enhancement after contrast injection.

3g. The centrum semiovale is a complex structure containing three systems of nerve fibers: the commissural system of the corpus callosum; the long and short association bundles between cortical areas in one hemisphere; and the projection fibers, both ascending from the thalamus and descending to basal ganglia, brainstem, and spinal cord. The latter group of fibers is sometimes referred to as corona radiata.

3h. The superior sagittal sinus, like the falx (see Question 3e), is cut across in two places in slice B: anteriorly (small diameter) and posteriorly (large, triangular diameter).

3i. The main tributaries to the straight sinus are the great cerebral vein of Galen and the inferior sagittal sinus (see Fig. 3.2 or Fig. 5.9B); others are the basal and cerebellar veins.

Chapter 4 4a. The posterior limb of the internal capsule (low density) is situated between two gray (high density) masses: the thalamus and the lentiform nucleus.

4b. The posterior limb of the internal capsule contains (ascending) thalamocortical, (descending) corticospinal, and some temporopontine fibers. The genu mostly contains corticobulbar fibers. The anterior limb contains frontopontine fibers and other systems.

4c. Three, even four, calcified (high-density) structures may normally be seen at the level of Figure 4.7: in the pineal gland, the glomus of the choroid plexus in each ventricular atrium, and, less frequently, the habenular commissure.

4d. Branches of the middle cerebral artery are found in the lateral fissure; the interhemispheric fissure contains branches of the anterior cerebral artery.

4e. The highest portion of the posterior fossa (infratentorial compartment) can just be seen in Figure 4.3, since the apex of the tentorium reaches quite high and thus may be cut in front of the posterior falx (see Fig. 2.2).

4f. All cerebral lobes are partially represented in slice C, as is the insula.

4g. The low-density crossing in CT images from left to right in front of the anterior horns is the genu of the corpus callosum. In spin echo MR images the genu has a low signal.

Chapter 5 5a. The two anterior cerebral arteries and some of their branches are found in the interhemispheric fissure, in front of the lamina terminalis.

5b. Parts of the frontal, temporal, and occipital lobes are seen in slice D (Fig. 5.3).

5c. Structures that form the wall of the inferior horn are the hippocampus and fimbria, choroid plexus and choroid fissure, tail of caudate nucleus, optic radiation fibers, and subcortical white matter. Most of these structures are supplied by the anterior choroidal artery.

5d. The thalamus lies immediately above, and the interpeduncular cistern lies just in front of the midbrain.

5e. The occipital lobe lies on the tentorium (cerebelli).

5f. All three cerebral arteries (middle cerebral artery, anterior cerebral artery, posterior cerebral artery) or their branches may be seen in contrast-enhanced scans at the level of slide D (Fig. 5.8).

5g. The middle cerebral artery is the most direct and largest continuation of the internal carotid artery; therefore, the incidence of emboli and metastases is higher in the territory of this vessel.

Chapter 6   6a. The following CSF spaces can be identified in Figures 6.11, 6.12, and 6.15A and B: lateral and third ventricles (without contrast); the subarachnoid space around the brain with its cisterns at the base of the brain; and the ambient and quadrigeminal cisterns (all with contrast).

6b. The major causes of subarachnoidal hemorrhage are rupture of an aneurysm; rupture of a superficial arteriovenous malformation; and complication of a subdural hemorrhage or an intracranial bleeding. Such subarachnoidal hemorrhages appear as high-density areas (60 to 100 Hounsfield units) in the cisterns on unenhanced CT images.

6c. The tips of the lateral (temporal) horns are curved and rather shallow because the hippocampus bulges into the ventricular space; usually they are not seen on 10-mm thick slices. An inferior horn that is clearly visible on CT indicates dilation, caused, e.g., by occlusion of the interventricular foramen (Monro's foramen) with subsequent enlargement of the entire ipsilateral ventricle, or by "entrapment" of the horn by a blocking mass.

6d. The optic nerve and chiasma have a CT density comparable to that of white matter (24 to 36 Hounsfield units), which is higher than the density of CSF (0 to 16 Hounsfield units).

6e. If the densities of the chiasma and CSF were alike (e.g., because of a small amount of blood in the cisterns), the outline of the chiasma could be shown by injecting air or iodinated contrast in those cisterns. This possibility is contraindicated in practice, because the contrast could cause severe and undesirable side effects. In a case of a recent subarachnoidal hemorrhage, contrast cisternography is unnecessary, is counterindicated, and does not make sense.

6f. Slice D contains portions of frontal, temporal, and occipital lobes.

6g. If the probable cause of the clinical syndrome is thought to be the rupture of a vessel or an intracranial bleeding, contrast injection is *contraindicated* since it would flow into or around an already damaged brain. If occlusion of a vessel is suspected, injection of contrast is usually not needed to make the diagnosis on a CT image (see Fig. 3.15).

Chapter 7   7a. Only the temporal lobe and the gyrus rectus of the frontal lobe are represented on slice F (Fig. 7.3B or 7.6).

7b. The intracavernous internal carotid artery and the intracranial internal carotid artery are seen twice in a coronal section because of the curvature of the siphon. The intracavernous internal carotid artery is shown more than once in Fig. 7.10B, since it has a tortuous course in this specimen (not uncommon in older patients).

7c. The lowermost gyrus of the frontal lobe seen in Figure 7.3 is the gyrus rectus.

7d. The CT density of the fourth ventricle is that of any CSF-containing space (0 to 16 Hounsfield units), and is lower than the density of the pons (a mixture of gray and white matter, 24 to 50 Hounsfield units).

7e. The sphenoid bone and air sinus lie just below the pituitary gland; the diaphragma sellae, stalk, chiasma, circle of Willis, and the suprasellar cistern lie just above the gland.

Chapter 8   8a. In a series of slices cut along the infraorbitomeatal base plane, the temporal lobe is represented more inferiorly than the frontal and occipital lobes; in other words, the middle cranial fossa lies deeper than the anterior cranial fossa and the tentorium (on which the occipital lobe rests).

8b. The upper halves of the orbits are separated by the ethmoid air cells, the lower halves by the nasal cavities.

8c. Within the internal auditory meatus are found cranial nerve VIII, cranial nerve VII with the nervus intermedius, and the auditory or labyrinthine artery. These structures are partially surrounded by CSF.

8d. The internal auditory meatus and labyrinth can be seen best on a series of thin, direct coronal or axial CT sections with bone window settings (see Fig. 8.12B). Another method for imaging the nerves entering the internal auditory meatus is illustrated in Figure 8.16A.

8e. The major components of the venous drainage of the brain visible in Figure 8.3 are the transverse sinus, the inferior petrosal sinus, and possibly the occipital sinus in the falx cerebelli (see Fig. 5.9).

8f. The paranasal sinuses seen in Figure 8.1A (both horizontal and parasagittal parts) are the frontal and sphenoidal air sinuses and ethmoid air cells. The maxillary air sinus lies in a lower axial plane.

8g. A purulent infection of the mastoid process (usually from an otitis media) can break through into the adjacent sigmoid sinus (see Fig. 8.4A), thus causing septicemia.

8h. Very wide window settings are best to display details of bone, e.g., sutures, fractures, etc.

Chapter 9   9a. The axis of each orbit diverges about 20° from the midsagittal plane, and lies in a plane approximately 10° angled down from the infraorbitomeatal base plane. Since the cone of muscles lies symmetrically around this axis, a true comparison between muscle sizes within each orbit requires a reformation at right angles to the orbital axis. To compare left and right orbit contents, sizes, and shapes, a series of reformations is needed (see Fig. 9.3).

9b. The optimal comparison between the thickness of one optic nerve with the other is made by obtaining two images, at right angles to each orbital axis, and then "flipping" one electronically, so that the configuration and diameters in each image are directly comparable.

9c. An infection of the face or nose may spread via the facial veins and ophthalmic veins to cause thrombophlebitis of the cavernous sinuses, resulting in a potentially life-threatening condition.

9d. The anastomoses between branches of the external carotid artery with branches of the ophthalmic artery (internal carotid artery branch) can serve as suppliers of arterial blood to parts of the brain in case of low internal carotid artery obstruction or occlusion. The anastomotic vessels may grow in size and the flow in the ophthalmic artery may become reversed.

9e. In the case of a sudden (traumatic) carotid-cavernous-fistula, the arterial pressure of the internal carotid artery is transmitted to the cavernous sinus and its tributaries; in the orbit, the ophthalmic veins (especially the superior ones) become considerably larger and may cause exophthalmus.

9f. The globes each rotate around a central point within the eye. In looking to the left, the posterior parts of each globe rotate to the right; in the right eye the optic papilla would therefore be more lateral (temporal). This can be demonstrated easily on CT images.

9g. Injection of contrast in the cisternal CSF (e.g., via a lumbar puncture plus downward tilting of the head) could be shown on CT to result in enhancement of the optic nerve sheath; in cases of increased cranial pressure the sheath would be enlarged, and papilledema may be demonstrable in the eye. (Of course, the latter could be more easily and cheaply demonstrated fundoscopically.)

Chapter 10   10a. The jugular foramen is partially divided by a bony spur into a pars nervosa and a pars vasculosa. The glossopharyngeus, vagus nerve, and spinal accessory nerves, as well as the sigmoid and inferior petrosal sinuses, pass through the foramen.

10b. The best procedure (using CT) to demonstrate the diameter of the cord is to inject contrast into the dural sac, and then obtain axial CT sections with a bone-window setting.

10c. A routine CT image of the craniovertebral junction is often degraded by streak-artifacts; moreover, soft tissues and sharply defined bone cannot be seen on the same image. An MR image does not show streak-artifacts.

10d. An intradural, extramedullary mass may be located in the subarachnoid space or in the subdural space, or in both.

10e. The strong transverse ligament contains the odontoid process of C2 close to the anterior arch of C1.

10f. There are several movements possible in the atlanto-occipital articulation. The main movement in the atlanto-axial articulation is anteroposterior extension and flexion ("nodding"), although other movements are also possible.

Chapter 11   11a. The main orientation of the articular facets in the cervical vertebrae (except C1 and C2) is in a left or right oblique coronal plane; the main orientation of the facets in the thoracic spine is in a coronal plane; flexion movements are thus readily possible, while lateral movements are limited.

11b. The functional importance of the cervical uncinate processes lies in the fact that lateral movement is limited while allowing anteroposterior movements; in conjunction with the orientation of the articular facets the uncinate processes provide good stability for the neck.

11c. The details of the intradural contents can best be visualized on CT images when there is contrast in the subarachnoid space (see Fig. 11.4).

11d. The spinal cord is largest in its (lateral) dimension at the cervical swelling, where the roots that form the brachial plexus course to or from the cord (C5 to T1). The vertebral canal (and the dural sac) are normally widest just below the foramen magnum (C1 level).

11e. Elevation of the arm may cause compression of the motor and sensory root in an ipsilateral intervertebral foramen between C5 and T1 when spondylosis or lateral osteophytes have caused narrowing of this foramen.

11f. In the C5-C6 intervertebral foramina the C6 spinal nerves are found; however, the T5 spinal nerves emerge from the T5-T6 intervertebral foramina.

Chapter 12

12a. The posterior aspect of the lumbar intervertebral discs is slightly concave, except for the L5-S1 disc, which is normally straight. Beginning herniations or protrusions of the nucleus pulposus may produce a flattened posterior margin of the intervertebral disc.

12b. The conus medullaris contains the lower lumbar, sacral, and coccygeal segments of the cord; the tip of the conus is found at the lower L1 or upper L2 vertebral level in adults. In children the conus is located on a lower level.

12c. A converging network of veins in the body of each vertebra (except C1) emerges posteriorly from the body, midway between the endplates by way of one or two basivertebral veins. These channels may mimic fractures. Large veins may resemble a bulging disc.

12d. The diarthrodial portion of the sacroiliac joint lies more inferiorly and anteriorly than the ligamentous portion; it is best distinguished and examined by oblique sections with gantry of the CT scanner tilted as suggested by Carrera and associates (Fig. 12.10).

12e. The location of the lower end of the spinal dural sac is best determined by injecting intrathecal contrast, and then examining it with radiologic methods such as myelography or CT; the presence of root cysts can be similarly documented.

12f. A herniated nucleus pulposus may extend posteriorly, posterolaterally, or far laterally through a cracked annulus fibrosus; a free fragment may move within the epidural space (usually downwards). A herniation may also occur upwards or downwards into the spongeous bone of the adjacent vertebral bodies and then form a so-called Schmorl's node.

Appendix A. Glossary of Terms, Abbreviations, and Acronyms

Abscess — A focus of suppuration within a tissue or organ

ACA — Anterior cerebral artery

ACoA — Anterior communicating artery

Adenocarcinoma — Malignant tumor of glandular epithelium

Adenoma — Benign tumor of glandular epithelium

AG — Angiogram; Angiography

AICA — Anterior inferior cerebellar artery

Algorithm — Multiple, complex calculations, such as those used to compute a CT image

ALS — Amyotrophic lateral sclerosis (Lou Gehrig's disease, motor neuron disease)

Alzheimer's disease — (Pre)senile dementia; degenerative cortical disease

Amipaque (Metrizamide) — Water-soluble contrast medium used in myelography

Aneurysm — (Local) ballooning or widening of blood vessel wall

Angulation — Angle of plane relative to infraorbital base plane

    Negative angulation: anteriorly downward

    Positive angulation: anteriorly upward

Anomia — Inability to recall names (form of aphasia)

Arteriosclerosis — Degenerative process in vessel wall, associated with calcium deposit and loss of elasticity, fatty degeneration, or ulceration and thrombus formation

Astrocytoma — Low-grade type of glioma

Atrophy — Loss of volume or bulk, associated with loss of function

AVM — Arteriovenous malformation (congenital or traumatic); one of the forms of vascular malformation

Axial — Referring to CT or MR plane that is approximately horizontal

BA — Basilar artery

Babinski's sign — Abnormal plantar reflex (toe up) indicative of "upper motor neuron" lesion

Bone window — Wide window setting

BP — 1) blood pressure; 2) bypass (graft)

Bruit — Murmur or sound over vessel, often related to turbulence, stenosis, or rapid flow

Bypass (graft) — A vascular/surgical procedure to improve circulation

CA — Cancer

Cancellous (diploic) bone — Spongy layer of bone between dense bone

CBC — Complete blood count. Normal erythrocyte count, 4.2 to 5.9 million/mm^3; normal leukocyte count, 4,800 to 10,800/mm^3; normal platelet count, 200,000 to 350,000/mm^3

CC — Carotid-cavernous (e.g., fistula)

Circumduction — Lateral swinging movement of leg in walking, associated with loss of flexor function

Clonus — Rapid, rhythmic muscle contractions after passive stretch

CN(N) — Cranial nerve(s)

Coarctation — Narrowing or stricture of a vessel, canal, or space

Commissure — Bundle of nerve fibers uniting similar structures in the two sides of the brain or spinal cord (see decussation)

Conray — Meglumine iothalamate, a contrast medium for intravenous urography or angiography

Contrast — The visual differentiability of variations in image densities (e.g., by contrast agent or contrast solution)

Contre coup — Injury opposite to the blow, e.g., on the skull

Convexity — Swelling or spherical form on the external surface

Corneals — Short for corneal reflexes (V1 to VIII)

Coronal — Pertaining to the crown (tiara) of the head (e.g., coronal suture or coronal plane)

Corona radiata — A radiating mass of white nerve fibers extending from the internal capsule to and from the cerebral cortex

Cortical ribbon — The continuity of cerebral cortex as seen in sections

CPA — Cerebellopontine angle

Craniopharyngioma — Infiltrative tumor, often cystic and with calcification

CRI — Cancer Research Institute

CRT — 1) Cranial radiation therapy; 2) Cathode ray tube

CSF — Cerebrospinal fluid

CT — Computed tomography: a method of imaging in which a computer is used to reconstruct the anatomic features recorded by x-ray tomography

CT density — Inherent quality of tissue, based on absorption of x-ray beam

CXR — Chest x-ray

Cysticercosis — Infection with larva of *Taenia solium* (tapeworm)

DDX — Differential diagnosis

Decubitis position — The recumbent or horizontal posture, supine or lateral

Decussation — A chiasma or "X"-shaped crossing of nerve fibers uniting dissimilar structures in the two sides of the brain or spinal cord (see Commissure)

Delay — Time interval between radio frequency excitation and receipt of signal in MR imaging (echo delay or echo time)

Dementia — Deterioration or loss of intellectual faculties, reasoning power, memory, and will due to organic brain disease

Demyelination — Loss of normal myelin

Density — X-ray attenuation in tissue

Digital-analog conversion — Change from digital computer information to analog computer information

Digital scan images — Obtained with CT, comparable to standard radiographs (see Scout view entry)

Diploe — Diploic bone. (see Cancellous bone)

Diplopia — Double vision

Disorientation x2, x3. Grades of inability to remember time, place, or person

DSA — Digital subtraction angiography

DTR — Deep tendon reflex(es)

DX — Diagnosis

Dysarthria — Inability to articulate words correctly (loss of function of lower cranial nerves)

Dysmetria — Inability to make coordinated movements over a certain distance, often with cerebellar dysfunction

ECA — External carotid artery

Echo delay — (see Delay)

Echo time (TE) — (see Delay)

Edema — Excessive accumulation of fluid in tissue

EDH — Extra(epi)dural hemorrhage

Effacement — Loss of form or features

Embolization — Therapeutic radiologic procedure by which abnormal vessels are reduced in size or occluded

EOM — Extraocular muscle movements

Ependymoma — A (glial) tumor made up of ependymal cells

Epidermoid — Cyst lined by epithelium

ER — Emergency room

ESR — Erythrocyte sedimentation rate, a measure of tissue destruction: normal rate: men, 1 to 13 mm/hour; women, 1 to 20 mm/hour

Etiology — The science or study of the causes of disease (often used as the "cause" of disease)

Exophthalmus — Abnormal prominence or protrusion of the eyeball

Forebrain (prosencephalon) — The anterior brain vesicle of the embryo that subdivides into telencephalon and diencephalon

FTN test — Finger to nose test used to test cerebellar coordination

FX — Fracture

Glioma — General term for tumors of glial tissue; several grades are recognized, from astrocytoma to glioblastoma (highly malignant)

GPE or GPEX — General physical exam

Gradients — Magnetic fields induced by gradient coils in an MR imaging instrument

Graves' disease — Disease of unknown cause associated with hyperthyroidism and exophthalmus

Gray scale — A scale indicating gradations in CT density from white (very dense) to black (no density); in MR imaging the meaning is different

HA — Headache

HAO — Hemianopia: a lesion in the visual pathways behind the chiasma

HCT — Hematocrit. Normal percentage: men, 42% to 50%; women, 40% to 48%

Hemiatrophy of the brain — Atrophy or reduction in size confined to one side of the brain, usually a congenital condition

Hemiparesis — Weakness of the extremity muscles on one side of the body

Hemorrhage — Bleeding

Hernia nuclei pulposi — Abnormal protrusion of the core of the intervertebral disc

Herpes encephalitis — A destructive, hemorrhagic infection of the brain, caused by the herpes simplex virus

Hexabrix — Contrast medium used in urography or angiography

Hgb — Hemoglobin. Men, 13 to 16 g/100 ml; women, 12 to 15 g/100 ml

Hounsfield units — Units of CT density

HT — Hypertension

HTS test — Heel to shin test used to test cerebellar coordination

HU — Hounsfield units

HX — History

Hydrocephalus — Distention of the cerebral ventricles with cerebrospinal fluid. Obstructive or noncommunicating: block in the CSF pathway from lateral ventricle to cisterna magna. Communicating: block in the CSF pathway between cisterna magna and sites of absorption in blood vessels

Hyperemia — Increased blood flow in a structure, resulting in distention of the blood vessels

Hypesthesia — Impairment of sensation

IAM — Internal auditory meatus

ICA — Internal carotid artery

ICP — Intracranial pressure

Incisura — A notch, fissure, or defect (incisura tentorii)

Infarct — A localized area of ischemic tissue necrosis due to inadequate blood flow

Intercurrent disease — A disease occurring during the course of another condition

Intrathecal — In the subarachnoid space, especially in the spinal cord

Inversion recovery mode — MR mode of imaging in which magnetization is first inverted by a pulse, then detected by a second pulse

IOMBP or IOMP or IOM — Infraorbitomeatal (base plane)

Kilogauss — Measure of magnetic strength (10 kilogauss = 1 tesla)

Lipoma — A benign tumor of adipose (fat) tissue

LLE — Left lower extremity

LP — Lumbar puncture

LUE — Left upper extremity

Mass effect — The change in position of brain structures caused by an intracranial mass (tumor, bleeding, abscess, etc.)

MCA — Middle cerebral artery

Medulloblastoma — A malignant cerebellar tumor in children

Melanoma — A malignant tumor of melanocytes

Meningioma — A usually benign tumor derived from arachnoid cells

Meningocele — A protrusion of the meninges through a defect in skull or spine, which is filled with CSF

Metastasis — Transfer of tumor to another site by way of the blood stream or lymph channels

Metrizamide (Amipaque) — A radiopaque diagnostic medium used in myelography or cisternography, or both

MG — Myelogram

Miosis — Constriction of the pupil

MMA — Middle meningeal artery

Modality — 1) A form of sensation, such as touch, pressure, vision, or audition; 2) also used as "technical procedure"

MR imaging — Imaging method using (Nuclear) Magnetic Resonance

MRI — see MR imaging

MS — 1) Multiple sclerosis; 2) mental status

Mucocele — An abnormal cystic structure filled with mucus

Mural nodule — A nodular cell mass in the wall of a cystic tumor

Nevus, naevus — Skin lesion containing melanine

NEX — Neurologic examination

NL (WNL) — Normal (within normal limits)

NMR — Nuclear magnetic resonance

N/V — Nausea/vomiting, often suggestive of rapid-growing intracranial mass

Nystagmus — Oscillary movement of the eyeballs. Spontaneous nystagmus is associated with vestibular lesions; nystagmus can be normally evoked

OD — 1) Overdose; 2) oculus dexter

OP — Opening pressure of LP. Normal pressure, 70 to 180 mm of water

OS — Oculus sinister

Osteoma — Usually benign tumor of bone tissue

Osteophyte — A bony outgrowth

Otitis media — Inflammation of the middle ear

Palsy — Paralysis or weakness, used to designate special types such as cerebral palsy, bulbar palsy, facial palsy

Paralysis — Loss of strength due to lack of innervation

Paresis — Weakness

Paresthesia — Abnormal sensations such as tingling, prickling, etc.; occurs with disease of the peripheral nerves, roots, or posterior columns of the spinal cord

PCA — Posterior cerebral artery

PCoA — Posterior communicating artery

PE — 1) Papilledema, seen by ocular funduscopy, sign of increased intracranial pressure; 2) pulmonary embolism

PEG — Pneumoencephalogram

PERRL — Pupils equally round and reactive to light

PEX — Physical examination

PICA — Posterior inferior cerebellar artery

Pinealoma — A tumor of the pineal gland; various types occur

Pixel — Picture element of an image derived from a scanned volume element or voxel

Plantar extensor — An abnormal reflex (in persons older than 2 years of age) indicating a lesion in the descending motor tracts

PMN — Polymorphoneutrophil (Polymorphonuclear leukocyte)

Porencephaly — Congenital defect extending from the surface of the cerebral cortex to the underlying ventricle

PR — Pulse rate (normally 60 to 80 pulsations per minute, depending on position of the body)

Proptosis — Exophthalmus, usually of one eye

Pt — Patient

PTA — 1) Prior to admission; 2) percutaneous transluminal angioplasty

Ptosis — Drooping of the upper eyelid (usually a sign of IIIrd nerve dysfunction)

Pulse — 1) Radiofrequency pulse used in MR imaging; 2) wave of vascular, dilatation detected in the wrist or elsewhere

PX — Prognosis

Quadriparesis — Weakness of all four limbs

Rad — Unit of absorbed radiation dose

RAM — Rapid alternating movements. Test for cerebellar function

RBC — Red blood cell count. Normal count: 4.2 to 5.9 million/ mm^3

Reconstruction — Reproduction by assemblage of serial sections

Reformation — Reconstruction from a series of CT images in one plane, of a computed image in a different plane

REM — Rapid eye movements (a stage of sleep)

Remission — Abatement of the symptoms of the disease

Repetition time — see TR

RF — Radiofrequency

RIND — Reversible ischemic neurological deficit (see TIA)

RR — Respiration rate. Normal rate: 12 to 18 per minute

RX — 1) Treatment; 2) prescription; 3) reflex

Sagittal plane — Median (midsagittal) or parallel to the median (parasagittal]

SAH — Subarachnoidal hemorrhage

SAS — Subarachnoid space

Scan — To observe systematically; also, a CT or MR image

SCbA — Superior cerebellar artery

Schwannoma — A usually benign tumor of the nerve sheath cells

Scotoma — An area of absent or depressed vision in the visual field, surrounded by an area of normal vision

Scout view — Digital radiograph of an anatomic region to be scanned

SDH — Subdural hemorrhage

Septicemia — Severe bacteremic infection, generally involving invasion of the microorganisms in the bloodstream

Serpiginous — Snake-like

Shunt — Artificial communication between CSF spaces or between a ventricle and body cavities or veins

Spina bifida — A congenital defect in the closure of the vertebral canal

Spin echo — MR imaging technique of excitation by RF pulse followed by a signal after an echo delay

Spondylosis — Stiffness or fixation of a vertebral joint, often due to degenerative bone growth

SS — Straight sinus

S/S — Signs and symptoms

SSS — Superior sagittal sinus

Stenosis — Narrowing of a lumen

Subhyaloid HR — Hemorrhage beneath the hyaloid membrane of the eye

Subluxation — Incomplete dislocation

Syndrome — Pattern of S/S typical for a disease entity

Syrinx — Abnormal, usually longitudinal, cavity within the spinal cord or brain stem

TE — Echo time or echo delay

T1 — Time constant (spin-lattice, or thermal, or longitudinal) relaxation time: a measure of tissue properties in MR imaging

T2 — Transverse (spin-spin) relaxation time: a measure of tissue properties in MR imaging

Thrombophlebitis — Inflammation of a vein associated with thrombosis

TIA — Transient ischemic attack (see RIND)

TR — Repetition time (pulse sequence interval): the time between repeated RF perturbations of a tissue volume

TSH — Thyroid stimulating hormone

Trabeculae — Bridging strands of tissue (e.g., in bone, in arachnoid)

VA — Vertebral artery

VDT — Video display terminal

Vector — Net magnetic moment (a term used in NMR)

Volume averaging — Distortion of a pixel density by scanning of a thick slice through structures of different CT densities

Voxel — Volume element

WBC — White blood cell count. Normal count: 4,800 to 10,800/ mm^3

Window width — An expression for "gating" of certain densities

WNL (NL) — Within normal limits

XRT — X-ray therapy

Appendix B. *General References*

Carrera, G. F., et al.: CT of sacroiliitis. A. J. R., *136*:41, 1981.

Chusid, J. G.: Correlative Neuroanatomy. 18th ed. Los Altos, Lange Medical Publications, 1982.

Cunningham's Textbook of Anatomy. 12th ed. Edited by G. J. Romanes. London, New York, Oxford University Press, 1981.

Escourolle, R., and Poirier, J.: Manual of Basic Neuropathology. Philadelphia, W. B. Saunders Co., 1971. Translated by L. J. Rubinstein.

Federle, M. P., and Brant-Zawadski, M. (eds.): Computed Tomography in the Evaluation of Trauma. Baltimore, Williams & Wilkins, 1982.

Gray's Anatomy. 35th British ed. Edited by R. Warwick, and P. L. Williams. Philadelphia, W. B. Saunders Co., 1973.

Kaufman, L., Crooks, L. E., and Margulis, A. R. (eds.): Nuclear Magnetic Resonance Imaging in Medicine. New York-Tokyo, Igaku-Shoin, 1981.

Malamud, N., and Hirano, A.: Atlas of Neuropathology. Berkeley and Los Angeles, University of California Press, 1974.

Margulis, A. R., et al.: Clinical Magnetic Resonance Imaging. Radiology Research and Education Foundation, University of California, San Francisco, and University Printing Department, 1983.

Mills, C. M., et al.: Nuclear Magnetic Resonance Imaging: Effect of Blood Flow. A. J. N. R. *4*:1161, 1983.

Moss, A. A. (ed.): NMR, Interventional Radiology, and Diagnostic Imaging Modalities. Department of Radiology, University of California, San Francisco, and University of California Printing Department, 1983.

Newton, T. H., and Potts, D. G. (eds.): Computed Tomography of the Spine and Spinal Cord. San Anselmo, Clavadel Press, 1983.

Newton, T. H., and Potts, D. G. (eds.): Advanced Imaging Techniques. San Anselmo, Clavadel Press, 1983.

Ralston, H. J.: Neuroanatomy: Clinical and Experimental. Philadelphia, Lea & Febiger. In preparation.

Unsöld, R., Ostertag, C. B., De Groot, J., and Newton, T. H.: Computer Reformations of the Brain and Skull Base. Berlin, Heidelberg, New York, Springer-Verlag, 1982.

Index

Page numbers in *italics* indicate figures; page numbers followed by "t" indicate tables.